How to Treat Your Dogs and Cats with Over-the-Counter Drugs Companion Edition

Robert L. Ridgway, DVM

Dr. Ridgway is the author of *How to Treat Your Dogs and Cats with Over-the-Counter Drugs*, eighteen professional journal articles, and five professional auto tutorials.

iUniverse, Inc.
Bloomington

How to Treat Your Dogs and Cats with Over-the-Counter Drugs Companion Edition

iUniverse books may be ordered through booksellers or by contacting:

iUniverse
1663 Liberty Drive
Bloomington, IN 47403
www.iuniverse.com
1-800-Authors (1-800-288-4677)

ISBN: 978-1-4697-7525-8 (sc)
ISBN: 978-1-4697-7523-4 (e)
ISBN: 978-1-4697-7524-1 (hc)

Library of Congress Control Number: 2012902568

Printed in the United States of America

iUniverse rev. date: 4/10/2012

To Gilbert W. Carl, DVM; Robert D. Pokorny, DDS;
Charles H. Beckmann, MD; Dan Johnson;
and all the men and women living and dead who have served our
nation in the United States Armed Forces from the American
Revolution onward.
If there be heroes, they have served our country honorably.

Contents

Foreword

You, the reader, should consider yourself extremely fortunate! You have picked up the definitive work on treating pets with over-the-counter drugs. It was written by a well-known veterinarian, Dr. Robert Ridgway, from Orlando, Florida. Dr. Ridgway has a wealth of experience treating dogs and cats, which he brings to you in this authoritative book. He has had a long, distinguished career as a practicing veterinarian, and he has a unique ability to transmit his knowledge—in easily understood terms—to readers like you and me.

Dr. Ridgway's early career was in the US Army, from which he retired as a lieutenant colonel. Much of his career was spent acquiring dogs for all the branches of the military. He traveled often to Germany, where his talents were put to good use in obtaining the best dogs possible. Following his military service, Dr. Ridgway entered private practice of veterinary medicine. He is now in practice in Orlando.

Dr. Ridgway is a very highly trained veterinarian. He received his doctorate degree in veterinary medicine from Kansas State University and thereafter completed a residency at the University of California. He is board-certified by the American College of Preventative Medicine and the American College of Laboratory Animal Medicine. Currently, Dr. Ridgway performs 450–500 surgical procedures per month. Clearly, he is a talented and experienced practitioner. Thus, he is uniquely qualified to transmit his vast knowledge in an easily readable manner to his readers.

As a practicing physician, I have found his insights and advice to be accurate, detailed, and immensely useful. His book gives me much useful information. Although I am a physician in practice, I found that I had a lot to learn about treating pets as compared to people. This book taught me all that I need to know. It is an excellent reference book that will be a valued part of my library.

This book is a companion to Dr. Ridgway's *How to Treat Your Dogs and Cats with Over-the-Counter Drugs*. It enlarges and expands on many new subjects and complements the original book very well. In addition to informing you on how to treat various conditions with over-the-counter medicines, this book tells you when to seek help from a veterinarian instead of treating at home. It also gives you excellent advice concerning prevention, which is an all-important topic that could save you much money!

This fine book is not meant to preclude timely visits to your favorite veterinarian. To his credit, Dr. Ridgway points out the conditions and circumstances that merit professional attention. For all of the above reasons, I am thrilled to add this valuable reference book to my library along with *How to Treat Your Dogs and Cats with Over-the-Counter Drugs*. I will refer to these two books often—and my pets will be all the better for it!

Charles H. Beckmann, MD, FACP, FACC, FAHA
Professor of Medicine, ret.
Uniformed Services University of the Health Sciences
Bethesda, Maryland, and San Antonio, Texas

Preface

This book is a companion to *How to Treat Your Dogs and Cats with Over-the-Counter Drugs*. It continues the premise of treating your pets with over-the-counter drugs, presenting additional guidance similar to that found in the companion book, *How to Treat Your Dogs and Cats with Over-the-Counter Drugs*. There are many conditions described that can be treated with over-the-counter drugs and many health conditions discussed that can be prevented if you are aware of the conditions and know what to do.

This book is about you and how you can treat your pet at home with the suggested treatment. It contains entirely different information from *How to Treat Your Dogs and Cats with Over-the-Counter Drugs*. Conditions are adequately, understandably, and simply described in common language and include—but are not limited to—conditions such as surgical site issues, euthanasia or humane death, bleeding wounds, identifying pain, oral warts, stings from insects, issues of the teeth, aged pets, and many more that occur frequently in cats and dogs of all ages and breeds.

The health conditions covered are those that occur in pets that often leave owners perplexed and feeling that they are not knowledgeable—or capable—enough to help their pet at home. In *How to Treat Your Dogs and Cats with Over-the-Counter Drugs*, the issues discussed, depending on your point of view, are perhaps a bit more basic and may be a bit more common than those covered in this book. If some issues are beyond an owner's ability due to lack of proper equipment or lack of over-the-counter drugs to treat some conditions, the pet's doctor may come into the treatment cycle. Each condition described has a provided treatment and a suggestion for preventing the health condition from occurring. Of course, it is best if we can prevent health issues from occurring; we are all pleased and happy to have healthy pets at the lowest cost—especially when it means a longer life for our pets. In addition to the many over-the-counter drug treatment suggestions, many preventive measures are described to help you keep your pet healthy from disease and trauma.

Most, if not all, of the issues described are seen every day and leave owners wanting for information. This is obvious from all the questions asked about pet conditions when seen by veterinarians. It is hoped that this book will help you identify issues and aid in the treatment of many common conditions at home with over-the-counter drugs and minimal fuss, allowing you to provide good health care for your pet.

I have noticed that many folks do not ever take their pet to see a doctor of veterinary medicine. Many do not have the financial means to do so; therefore, the pet's health suffers. Furthermore, many people purchase over-the-counter drugs and give their pets an overdose, making pets sick or even killing the pet by trying to help their little buddy. This book aids all those who have these types of issues—and even those who do not. These three reasons are the stimulus for publishing these books to help you overcome these types of issues. If the suggestions are followed, I know your pet's health will be greatly enhanced.

Obviously the treatment and preventions are only suggestions; there may be additional methods that are just as effective. It is not the intent of this book to list every treatment and prevention that is available; it is meant to provide to you with a simple, straightforward approach to treating your pet with over-the-counter drugs. This book provides you with a means to aid your pet's health with over-the-counter drugs. This is not a first-aid book—this is a how-to-do-it-yourself book to aid you in maintaining your pet's health at home with over-the-counter drugs.

The book provides proper dosages, how many days to give the drug, and where the over-the-counter drug can be purchased at local pharmacies, grocery stores, Wal-Mart, Petco, and PetSmart stores in your community.

I am most happy that you think enough of your pet to purchase this book to help you keep your pet healthy and living a long, healthy life. You must understand that you alone make decisions to use and follow suggestions for over-the-counter drugs. Neither the publisher nor I can be responsible for your improper use of drugs or unexpected drug reactions that can—and do—occur. We are not present to aid in your diagnosis and treatment decisions; you alone bear responsibility for your pet and your pet's health. Here is to you and your pet's health as you launch your home health program. Remember that it is best to take your pet to see your pet's doctor for all health conditions. However, since we know that may not always be possible, use this guide. If you have questions and/or suggestions for inclusions in any future publications, please send a message to dogcatotc@gmail.com. We would love to hear from you—good or bad. Good luck to you and your healthy pet always.

Chapter 1:
Trauma

One should avoid an unfamiliar word as a ship avoids a reef.
—Julius Caesar

Here we will discuss issues that perhaps could have—and should have—been avoided. Life happens quickly, and we wonder how in the world our pet could become so severely traumatized. Many trauma occurrences are the result of a lack of thinking. Or we think all is well, and we ignore or don't properly supervise our pets—or we let them out alone. Maybe we walk them with without a leash. When the unexpected happens so quickly, even a quick reaction cannot always prevent an accident. We will discuss several conditions that you can care for with over-the-counter drugs. We also provide you with a suggestion for how you can prevent things from occurring or reccurring.

When Surgical Sutures Fail (Dehiscence)

On occasion, traumatic events occur. A pet may constantly chew at a surgery site, causing the sutures to come undone. If it happens to be a major body cavity, there is always a chance that internal organs may be discharged through the hole in the suture line. Most often, there is a swelling under the skin incision. It is not uncommon to see a collection of fluid (seroma) or tissues that do not belong in

1

that position. Tissues under the incision may mean the surgery has ruptured and internal organs are trying to exit. If you happen to see an unusual swelling under *any* suture line within the first ten days of surgery, it needs to be accessed as soon as possible. Let your pet's doctor be the one who determines what needs to be done. Delay can result in strangulation of organs or a body cavity infection.

Treatment:

If your pet is licking or chewing at any surgery site, you need to get an Elizabethan collar (E-collar) to keep the pet from destroying the surgery site. E-collars are available at PetSmart and Petco. Do not delay—get one fast. If you do not get an E-collar and the incision comes open for any reason, get your pet back to the facility that did the surgery as fast as possible. It is normally very easy to tell that the pet has been chewing at the suture line. Do not lie to your pet's doctor about how it came undone. Delay can be dangerous; this should be considered an emergency.

The pet needs to be returned to the facility that performed the surgery for a proper evaluation of a sub-skin swelling or an open surgery site as soon as possible. Delay in returning for evaluation normally results in greater tissue damage than is necessary. If it happens to be a seroma, the fluid can be very easily drained. If it is tissues under the skin, you will not be able to tell the difference. Let the doctor be the determiner of the condition—and do not delay. A delay may be the cause of the death of your pet.

Although sutures may come undone (dehiscence), this is very rare unless you let your pet chew at the incision. Be aware that this can—and does—happen. Be prepared to take quick, appropriate actions. Unfortunately, many folks ignore a pet chewing at a surgery site and wait until it is destroyed before returning to the doctor. You do not need the extra expense of letting your pet destroy a surgery line. Get an E-collar for your pet.

Prevention:

As soon as you see any problem with the pet chewing at any surgery site, get an E-collar or take your pet to see the pet's doctor. Delay is not wise.

Bleeding or Hemorrhage

There are numerous causes of bleeding in pets, from obvious and easily seen issues to unseen diseases, such as intestinal bleeding. These can cause loss of blood in pets. We will discuss only those we can observe—signs that alert us to the fact that the pet has a bleeding problem.

The most obvious is skin trauma—the sort that cuts blood vessels—resulting in little to massive loss of blood. The amount of blood lost depends on the types of blood vessels that are ruptured or cut. A little blood can look like the Battle of the Bulge, but it may be a very small amount of blood. A common issue is the panic that owners have when a pet is bleeding.

It is important to count to ten and keep your cool so you can function and stop the pet's loss of blood. Bleeding from the legs, chest, abdomen, head, or other parts needs to be stopped as soon and as efficiently as possible. Bleeding from the nose is difficult to stop. Most of the time, nose bleeding is from a small blood vessel within the nose. Petechial bleeding (pin-sized hemorrhage spots on the skin) can be recognized by the little spots in the skin. The spots are normally widespread—the little red dots look somewhat like measles. This type of bleeding is the result of Rocky Mountain spotted fever or metabolic disorders, such as a lack of platelets in the blood. Platelets are important in the process of promoting clotting of blood.

Treatment:

The most important thing to do is keep calm and not panic. Panicking could result in the death of your pet due to your lack of ability to handle the situation. In most cases, the best action is to consider how to slow the bleeding and take your pet to the veterinary clinic as soon as possible. Of course, if it is minor bleeding, you will be able to treat and stop the bleeding yourself. This is similar to treating yourself when you cut yourself.

If a leg has been cut off, apply a tourniquet to stop the bleeding. The best action to take is to apply pressure to the bleeding area. Any deep blood vessels will be more difficult to get the bleeding to stop.

There is a product called PetClot available online at http://www.drugstore.com or http://www.quikclot.com. If you use the QuikClot website, click on "Shop for QuikClot," and then click on PetClot. These over-the-counter products are good for stopping bleeding fast. You may be aware that similar products are available. QuikClot has a product designed to stop nose bleeding. Remove the PetClot from the package, apply with pressure to the wound, and the bleeding will stop fast. PetClot is ideal for treating larger pets and farm animals. This product is very effective; however, one has to have it on hand for emergencies. The product cost is relatively low. It is a good product to have on hand for such an occasion. Follow the directions on the package.

Even though you can see petechial bleeding on the skin, this syndrome is definitely beyond your ability to diagnose and treat. Most often, it will require tests of some sort to get a diagnosis before the condition can be treated. Be cautious. If you cause additional pain, your pet might bite you as you try to treat the bleeding. Many pet owners have been bitten while helping their pets. You can tie the mouth shut before working on your pet if you think you might be bitten. I have suffered more than one bite—it is better to be safe than hurting and wishing you had tied the mouth shut.

Prevention:

It may be trite to say, but keeping good control of your pet can prevent bleeding. Don't allow your pet to be in areas without proper supervision.

Oh No, Broken Bones

Many pets manage to be the recipient of powerful trauma that breaks a bone—or bones. Those who fix bones can tell, in many cases, what the animal was attempting to do by the type of fracture. The most common fracture is a leg, followed by pelvis and back fractures. Head fractures are rare in our facility. Of course any bone in the body can be fractured.

When a traumatic event occurs, the animal is in pain. When attempting to aid an injured animal, many people get bitten—sometimes quite badly. Be conscious of the fact that they are hurt; if you do something that makes them hurt more, they may bite. If it is possible to get the pet to an emergency hospital or clinic quickly, then little needs to be done other than to comfort the animal and go. The veterinarian will be able to treat pain, stop bleeding, and perhaps stabilize the fracture until surgery can be performed. However, if this cannot be done, you can take some measures yourself. If you will not take the pet to the veterinarian, you can still help.

Treatment:

If the fracture happens to be the lower front or back leg, you can apply a Robert Jones splint. You will need a roll of cotton tape and an Ace bandage. Apply tape to the front of the leg and the back of the leg and extend the tape well beyond the foot—perhaps the length of the distance between the elbow and the foot or the hock to the foot. On a large dog, use a whole roll of cotton. On smaller dogs, half a roll will suffice. After you have the tape in place and significant distance of tape below the foot, start wrapping the cotton around the leg. When you have half a roll on the leg, take the long strands of tape and pull the front tape up over the cotton on top of the leg and the bottom stand of tape up behind the leg and then continue to wrap the cotton. Keep the foot below the cotton and make sure you can see the foot. The tape will help keep the splint from slipping down.

After the roll of cotton is on the leg, apply the Ace bandage. Wrap the bandage around the cotton roll as tightly as you can—and cover the entire roll of cotton. Then tape the end of the Ace bandage when you have finished wrapping the Ace bandage around the cotton on the leg. You should be able to thump the rolled cotton and tape and it should sound like you are thumping a watermelon. This is a good splint; as long as you keep it dry, it will keep the leg stable. If the dog has a broken back, it may never walk again—and the dog needs to be handled very carefully. If you suspect a broken back, it is best to place the pet on a hard surface for transporting. Make sure no more trauma occurs while handling the pet. Remember cats and dogs bite if you hurt them—be cautious. Ribs and other bones are difficult to stabilize. You will need to handle the pet carefully and keep it as calm as possible until you can obtain professional help.

Prevention:

The primary cause of broken bones in pets is from being hit by a car. This trauma is most often due to owners allowing their pets out without a leash or supervision, which allows the pet to get into the street and be hit by a car. If you love your pet, why take the chance of letting it loose without you and a leash? Be wise—not sad. Why invite unnecessary expenses by having to go to the pet's doctor to have bones fixed?

Achilles Tendon Injury

An achilles tendon injury can be easily identified because the hock drops down and the dog is lame on the injured rear leg. There are many causes of injuries to the three tendons of the achilles tendon. Too often, many owners do not have this condition treated. Lack of treatment causes the poor dog to be crippled. This normally requires surgery, but if you do not intend to have a veterinarian treat the pet, you can do the following treatment. The prognosis with home treatment is unknown.

Treatment:

At the minimum, a splint can be applied to the leg. It is important that the splint is examined frequently to prevent skin sores. If you make a homemade splint, be sure to pad it well to prevent more damage. Make sure the leg is in what would be the normal position of the leg at all times. This could be a permanent arrangement. On occasion, the tendon might heal if you have the leg properly positioned—and if you apply the splint very shortly after the injury. An issue with splinted legs is that the pet cannot properly use the leg, resulting in severe muscle disuse. With muscle atrophy, the leg becomes skinnier until the muscles disappear.

In addition to muscle atrophy, the joints suffer from disuse. Physical therapy becomes necessary to enable the use of the leg if the splint is removed. Be aware of long-term splinting of extremities for any pet. A trip to the pet's doctor may be the best thing you can do. The pet's doctor can be a big help with this issue.

Prevention:

Achilles tendon issues are the result of trauma of some sort; prevention is the key to this issue.

Stings from Bees, Wasps, Hornets, and Ants

More dogs than cats get stung by insects. You may not see the animal get stung, and the lesions may look like an allergic response. There may be swelling, or the dog may be exhibiting pain. Examine the dog carefully, and you may find the stinger. If possible, pull it out carefully because the top of the stinger has a little sack that contains venom. If you squeeze it, you will inject more venom into your pet and cause more pain.

Ants cause little red welts, and normally several welts are present (unlike a bee, wasp, or hornet sting). After a period of time, the ant bites may turn black. This can be seen on the belly of the dog, where there is less hair. Other insects will cause similar appearances on the belly skin.

Treatment:

The treatment is a dose of diphenhydramine (Benadryl). You can obtain Benadryl at grocery stores, drugstores, and Wal-Mart. The appropriate dosage varies, depending upon the size and weight of the pet. You can give .4 mg per pound of body weight or 1 mg per kilogram (2.2 pounds) of body weight for a low dose or .8 mg per pound or 2 mg per kg of body weight for a higher dose. Benadryl dose charts are below.

Benadryl 1 and 2 mg
First-Dose Chart Available Over-the-Counter in Grocery Stores
(Repeat Dose if Necessary)

	Dose 1 mg tablets	Weight Pounds	Dose 2 mg tablets
1	1/4 or 25	1	See 1 mg dose
2	1/2 or 5	2	See 1 mg dose
3	1	3	See 1 mg dose
4	1.5	4	See 1 mg dose
5	1.75	5	See 1 mg dose
6	2	6	1
7	3	7	1.5
8	3	8	1.5
9	4	9	2
10	4	10	2
11	5	11	2.5
12	Do not use	12	3
13	Do not use	13	3
14	Do not use	14	3.5
15	Do not use	15	3.5
16	Do not use	16	4
17	Do not use	17	4
18	Do not use	18	4
19	Do not use	19	5
20	Do not use	20	5

Benadryl 25 Mg First Dose Chart
Available Over-the-Counter in Drugstores
(Repeat Dose if Necessary)

Weight Pounds	Dose * # of tablets	Weight Pounds	Dose # of tablets	Weight Pounds	Dose # of tablets	Weight Pounds	Dose # of tablets
21	.5	41	1	61	2	81	2
22	.5	42	1	62	2	82	2
23	.5	43	1	63	2	83	2
24	.5	44	1	64	2	84	2
25	1	45	1	65	2	85	2
26	1	46	1	66	2	86	2
27	1	47	1	67	2	87	2
28	1	48	1	68	2	88	2
29	1	49	1	69	2	89	2
30	1	50	1	70	2	90	2.5
31	1	51	1.5	71	2	91	2.5
32	1.25	52	1.5	72	2	92	2.5
33	1.25	53	1.5	73	2	93	2.5
34	1.25	54	1.5	74	2	94	2.5
35	1.25	55	1.5	75	2	95	2.5
36	1.25	56	1.5	76	2	96	2.5
37	1.25	57	1.5	77	2	97	3
38	1.25	58	1.5	78	2	98	3
39	1.25	59	2	79	2	99	3
40	1.25	60	2	80	2	100	3

*1=1 tablet, .25 = 1/4 tablet, .5 = 1/2 tablet, .75 = 1/2 + 1/4 tablets.

Prevention:

Owners need be aware of a hostile environments in which their pet exercises to enable owners to to prevent deadly exposure to ant, bees, wasp and hornets. Negligence on an owner's part can result in either injury or death of the pet due to anaphylaxis, which causes constriction of the smooth muscles of the lungs. If the lungs collapse, the collapse will prevent breathing. Bees or wasps can start a big hive in bushes; in such cases, the numbers of stingers is excessive. Get those hives removed. We had one in our yard that was larger than a man's head. We were not even aware it was present, but it was very dangerous. The hive was removed by a professional bees' nest remover. Be aware of the possibility of bees and wasps and avoid obvious stinging insects, such as ants.

Collapse

Collapse is caused by loss of normal coordination functions of muscles that support the body. There are many syndromes and types of trauma that will cause an animal to collapse. Overexertion is perhaps one of the simplest to overcome that tends to occur most frequently in overweight dogs. A pet may collapse during exercise or while hunting. Signs of impending collapse might include the pet slowing down, weakness, unwillingness to get up, anxiety, vomiting, diarrhea, respiratory distress, and often increased respiratory rate. Although many systemic health conditions can cause collapse, such as heart problems, diabetes, heat, and other diseases, they require a a veterinarian to determine what caused the collapse.

Treatment:

You must determine the cause of the pet's collapse. However, once you feel comfortable that heat or overexertion was the cause of the collapse, get the animal inside. Keep it warm if due to exertion. If the collapse is due to heat exhaustion, cool your pet down with cool running water. Your pet should respond to your treatment within an hour and a half. If you determine that the cause of collapse is due to exertion or overexcitement, you can give your pet one or two tablespoons of Karo syrup. Keep the animal calm and offer small amounts of water if the animal is up. If you are unsure of the cause of the collapse, you need to take your pet to see the pet's doctor as soon as possible because this can be a life-threatening event. The key to successful treatment of the simple collapse discussed here is recognizing that the animal is in trouble and stopping whatever activity you have the pet participating in and start your treatment as soon as possible.

Prevention:

A wellness plan from your pet's favorite doctor is the best prevention you can have for collapse and many other syndromes. Knowing the health status of your pet goes a long way toward deciding what might be the cause of the collapse. Do not run your pet on extremely hot days—this is a sure way to kill a dog. We experienced a person riding a bicycle on a hot day with his dog running alongside. All of a sudden, the dog dropped like a rock—its body temperature was out of sight, and the dog died. You might think it is expensive to enroll in a wellness program for your pet; however, it is much cheaper to pay for a wellness visit than for the treatment of any health issue. Semiannual physicals or health checks help extend the life of your pet—as well as keeping you abreast of your pet's health status.

Gunshot Wounds

Gunshot wounds are definitely a job for your dog's doctor. However, there are some things you should know about gunshot wounds. Since the entry hole is usually smaller than the exit, it is normally easy to determine the direction of travel of the bullet. You would be surprised at the large numbers of dogs with a load of buckshot in the back end—particular hunting dogs. The direction of the buckshot is determined by the heavy load of buckshot as it thins out quickly forward of the entry level. Wounds can be in the legs, chest, or belly. With high-powered pistols and rifles, the bullet most often goes through the body. Radiographs or X-rays can be taken to see the conditions caused by the bullet or buckshot.

If a bullet penetrates the abdominal cavity, radiographs will not be of much benefit because the abdominal cavity is all soft tissue. Soft tissues do not show on radiographs. However, radiographs will sometimes show air in the abdominal cavity and excessive air in the guts. The intestines will have received considerable damage that may require cutting out sections of the gut to fix. Due to the close looping and back-and-forth construction of the intestines, the number of times the intestine is penetrated is normally excessive. There are usually several entry and exit points throughout the intestines. The holes in the intestines allow intestinal contents into the abdominal cavity and cause infections in the abdominal cavity (peritonitis) rather quickly.

If the chest is penetrated and the heart and major blood vessels are not hit, the chest will normally be full of air and the bullet will carry hair into the wound. It has not proven worthwhile to open a gunshot wound to remove the hair. Radiographs are of great benefit for chest wounds. With all the air that gets into the chest, many things that are not normally seen are easily seen due to the large amount of air in the chest cavity. There may be soft tissue wounds or shattered bones. Radiographs are a big aid for limb gunshot wounds, but each case is different.

Treatment:

Normally the dog will require extensive nursing care. The primary treatment is to stop bleeding and evaluate the extent of the damage. Your dog's doctor will have the equipment, anesthesia, and other articles necessary to treat your pet. It may also be necessary to make a decision to treat or to euthanize. PetClot is a great product for stopping bleeding; simply apply the gauze material next to the wound and apply pressure. However, one has to have the PetClot available to use. It is inexpensive and easy to carry on a hunting trip. You can purchase PetClot at www.petclot.com.

Prevention:

Some hunters get angry at their dog and blast it with a load of shot. Rather than shoot the dog in the rear, count to ten, keep your cool, and do not shoot the dog. Treat the dog as if it is your best buddy. Other types of ammunition tend to cause considerably more damage and firearm safety is always the best practice. Many pet buddies are accidently shot when crossing a fence or while performing some other maneuver. When getting into a shelter or a chair in a tree, don't point the weapon in an odd direction—and keep the safety on.

Broken or Fractured Teeth

There was a time in the past when broken or fractured teeth were ignored. Most teeth were pulled if they were broken or chipped. In this millennium, we have advanced beyond this type of treatment. That is the good news. The bad news is that there is very little an owner can do for fractured or broken teeth. Anesthesia is usually required to work on teeth—even to pull a tooth—unless it is so rotten that it is about to fall out. Rotten teeth are most often due to soft food diets. The food cakes on the teeth and aids in tooth decay.

Treatment:

Broken teeth prevention is the way to go. Providing really hard items, such as bones, ice cubes, nylon toys, cow hooves, and rocks, is the main cause of many broken or fractured teeth. The other cause of bad teeth is not cleaning them. Use products that help keep teeth clean, brush the teeth, or have routine cleanings—just as you do for yourself. Choose toys and food that allow for decreased plaque and calcium accumulation without fracturing teeth.

Prevention:

It is common to offer a dog rawhide, large bones, or other items from pet stores, but many will—and do—cause trauma to teeth. It is best to avoid these, as they are the cause of many broken teeth. As for tooth decay, ProDen PlaqueOff™ has been shown to be effective against bad breath, tartar, and plaque for animals. The product can be obtained by calling (909) 646-9949 or by going online to www.tartarshield.com.

Chewing on Extension Cords or Electrocution

Chewing on electrical cords occurs most commonly in kittens and puppies during the holiday season. Many exposed electrical cords and lines may be present in the house during holiday periods.

Chewing on electrical cords can cause complications such as burns or death—or it may be nothing more than a shock to the pet. Most commonly, burns in the mouth are quite painful and may require supplemental feeding via stomach tubes. The lungs and heart can also be involved. Diagnosing these syndromes will require the help of your friendly veterinarian. You can tell if the mouth or lips have been burned by the electrical cords.

Treatment:

If you have pets under the age of one and a half, the probability of them chewing on electric wires is higher. Limit the number of cords and keep them out of the way as much as possible. Frequently there is no trauma or very minor trauma due to the shock. Look at the pet to see if it is having difficulty breathing or if it has collapsed. There is a good chance the lungs or the heart has been involved. If so, the pet will need professional help. If the mouth is burned, antibiotics may be required. The extent of medical treatment will depend on the severity of the trauma.

Prevention:

Be aware. Keep cords in such a way that your pets cannot get to them.

Blood under the Ear Skin or Ear Hematoma

The cause of this syndrome is normally a combination of issues that are the result of lack of proper care of the pet's ears, which results in either the pet shaking their head a lot or excessive scratching at the ears. Cats do not have ear hematomas as frequently as dogs. However, it tends to be more common in cats that do a lot of scratching at their ears. The most common cause of head shaking or scratching at the ears is an infestation of ear mites that is left untreated. The lack of treatment of ear mites can—and does—lead to ear infections, which can be very difficult to treat and maintain a healthy ear.

Flop-eared or pendulous-eared dogs are more prone to ear infections and ear hematomas. Infestation of ear mites and infections causes pets to shake their heads a lot, which causes the ears to be whipped somewhat like a towel that has been shaken hard. The shaking puts pressure on the ear, causing the skin on the ear to separate from the underlying cartilage. The separation of the skin from the cartilage occurs on the same side of the ear as the opening to the ear canal. The separation of skin from the cartilage causes bleeding into the space between the ear skin and cartilage, resulting in an accumulation of blood under the skin. This is more commonly called an ear hematoma.

Treatment:

The best treatment is prevention. Just make sure the ears are clean and free of ear mites. It is a good idea to have a preventive medicine program or a wellness program. Have your dog looked at every six months by the pet's doctor to assure that the pet is in good health. A little preventive medicine saves a lot of money for owners. It may not seem so at the time, but paying for prevention is much cheaper than paying for treatments.

At home, do routine exams of the ears and ear cleaning to be sure there are no ear mites. Problems occur when pet owners do not look at the ears and are unaware of potential ear problems. When least expecting a health issue and without notice, the pet starts scratching at the ear and shaking the head. If a pet gets an ear hematoma, then the treatment is normally beyond the control of the owner; the dog will need to see the veterinarian. Without treatment, the ears tend to contract and form a cauliflower ear formation that does not look good on any pet.

Prevention:

Look at the ears often and keep the ears clean. If they become dirty, they should be cleaned. A WaterPik is an excellent tool for cleaning pet ears. It is best to use a straight tip on the WaterPik. You can make one by cutting the end of a bent tip. If you use a WaterPik, use warm water. The WaterPik is very effective and easy to use. A WaterPik can be purchased at drugstores or at Costco. A wellness program is highly recommended. See your pet's doctor and get it set up.

Never Leave a Pet Alone in a Vehicle

Leaving a pet in a vehicle—even with the windows cracked—makes one think that the car will not heat up. Even if the window is down an inch or two, you could not be more wrong. Heat has short and long wavelengths. Short heat waves penetrate glass, but long heat waves do not. As a short heat wave passes through glass, the short wave is converted to a long, low-energy heat wave and because it is unable to penetrate glass (actually glass reflects the low-energy long heat wave), the heat wave stays within the vehicle, causing heat to accumulate and a rapid temperature increase.

If outside temperatures are from 72–96 degrees, the temperature will rise at a rate of 1.9 degrees per minute in the first ten minutes inside the vehicle. As time passes, the temperature inside the vehicle increases faster—even though the rate of increase per minute decreases. After thirty minutes, temperatures can be thirty degrees higher than the outside temperatures. Thus, an outside temperature of 91 can cause the inside vehicle temperatures to reach a temperature of 120 degrees. Left ten minutes more, temperatures can reach near 130 degrees. In an hour, it can be close to 145 degrees.

Treatment:

The best treatment is not allowing the pet to be left alone in a vehicle. A thermometer and fan are essential tools for treatment of overheated pets. If possible, a cool treatment room is very beneficial. The most important thing is to get the body temperature down by putting cool water (not ice water) on the pet and turning a fan on the pet if available. Take the temperature frequently to see if you are progressing with the cooling of the body temperature. The fan helps the cooling process.

Temperatures of a pet left in a car can be above 107 degrees— and it is very difficult to get body temperatures down when the pet gets that hot. I have seen temperatures so high that the thermometer would not record the temperature. This is not a five-minute treatment; it is tedious to get body temperatures down. Success can be yours if you persist.

If after a prolonged period you are unsuccessful in getting body temperature down, the prognosis becomes grave. Remember that cold ice will cause surface blood vessels to constrict in response to cold. Putting ice on an overheated pet is a common mistake.

Prevention:

To prevent heat exhaustion or killing your family companion, do not leave your pet alone in a vehicle. This syndrome happens way too often—do not let it happen to you.

Do not leave pets unattended in any vehicle—at any time. If you know you will be parking your vehicle and you have to leave your pet in the vehicle, leave the pet at home.

Emergencies Not Treatable with Over-the-Counter Drugs

The following animal conditions are considered to be veterinary emergencies that need the attention of your pet's doctor for consultation and/or treatment. These conditions should be considered beyond your ability to treat. These conditions have been identified by the American Veterinary Medical Association as pet emergencies needing professional consultation and/or treatment:

a. Severe bleeding or bleeding that does not stop within five minutes

b. Choking, difficulty breathing, nonstop coughing, or gagging

c. Bleeding from the nose, mouth, rectum, coughing up blood, or blood in the urine

d. Inability to urinate or pass feces (stool), or obvious pain associated with urinating or passing stool

e. Eye injuries

f. Suspicion that your pet has eaten something poisonous (antifreeze, xylitol, chocolate, rodent poison, etc.)

g. Seizures or staggering

h. Fractured bones, severe lameness, or inability to move a leg

i. Obvious signs of pain or extreme anxiety

j. Heat stress or heatstroke

k. Severe vomiting or diarrhea—more than two episodes in a twenty-four-hour period (or either of these combined with obvious illness or any of the other problems listed here)

l. Refusal to drink for twenty-four hours or more

m. Unconsciousness

Treatment:

Many things that happen to pets require consultation and/or treatment by veterinarians. The purpose of this book—and *How to Treat Your Dogs and Cats with Over-the-Counter Drugs*—is how to treat your pet. There are some conditions that just do not fall into the treat-it-yourself category; for the health of the pet, it is necessary to seek professional help. However, there is a new product that will stop bleeding fast. PetClot is available online at http://www.drugstore. com/QuikClot or www.petclot.com. The good news is that it is rather inexpensive. But, to be effective, you must have it on hand.

Prevention:

The best prevention is to seek out a wellness program that your veterinarian provides and to have routine checks on a scheduled basis throughout the year for the life of your pet. So many things on the list above are caused by owners letting pets out without supervision and expecting the animal to come home on its own, but they could not be more wrong.

Be a buddy to your pet. Take the time to be outdoors with your pet. I have been called out so many times at two or three in the morning because of poisoning or a pet receiving trauma. I know that proper supervision of a pet outdoors pays big, big dividends. Just do it—and it will save you money and heartburn big time.

Areas of Missing or Denuded Skin

Unfortunately, trauma can cause skin to be removed or denuded from different areas of the body that needs skin to grow back or to be replaced. There are multiple options for fixing the denuded area by surgery, skin grafts, or closing skin over the area. This discussion will focus on the smaller areas that you can treat. How the skin was removed is not important. What is important is that we get skin to grow back in the areas denuded of skin. For treatment of smaller areas of missing skin, you will need to gather nonadherent dressing items, gauze sponges, either two-by-two or four-by-four inch gauze pads, and tape to hold the bandage.

Treatment:

For areas where the skin is missing that are easy to bandage, apply a moist gauze bandage to the wound; cover it with the nonsticking-type bandage, such as a telfa pad; wrap the entire bandage with a few rounds of gauze; and then tape the bandage in place so it will not slip down. Change the bandage frequently. With this treatment, the skin will grow into the denuded area. Unfortunately, it will not grow back overnight. Be patient and persistent with the moist bandage and with daily bandage changes. In time, you will have a healed wound. If you are unwilling to change the bandage daily, do not use this procedure, as the bandage must be clean and moist at all times for this procedure to work. Your patience and persistence will pay off, and your pet will thank you for your efforts.

Prevention:

The best prevention of trauma is to keep your pet on a leash at all times when you take your pet out. I have been called out numerous times because some owner turned his or her dog out in the early morning—and the pet was hit by a car. This is totally avoidable by owners recognizing the issues of a pet running loose in the neighborhood. These pets are a part of the family—would you turn your child loose? Heavens no! Do not turn your pet loose—the consequences are death or serious trauma, which hit the pocketbook big time.

Chapter 2:
From Birth to Six Months of Age

Do what you can, with what you have, where you are.
—Theodore Roosevelt

In this chapter, we will learn about newborn puppies and kittens and what to expect as they develop. As they grow, you need to evaluate the young to make sure that their growth is healthy and proper and that they are developing properly. It is amazing how quickly things can go wrong if you are not on top of development of the young. Simple things that you may never have given thought to will be discussed. If you follow the simple processes in this chapter, you will raise healthy, happy animals. Here is to the young who have you to look forward to for their future.

Puppies and Kittens Younger Than Four Weeks of Age

Newborn cats and dogs sleep and nurse frequently. Body weight change is very important to monitor to assure good health. Failure to gain weight in a few days is a sign of poor health in the young. Body weight should be monitored at birth, at twelve hours of age, and daily for the first two weeks. Newborn pups and kittens can be identified by characteristic coloring or markings or by using marker collars or ribbons of different colors. Use your own idea—as long as you can identify the same one over and over for the next few weeks.

You can record weight gain on the pages provided at the back of this book. Record weight gain and note if there is no gain; failure to gain weight is often the first sign of illness in a newborn kitten or puppy.

Treatment:

I suggest a gram scale. Some diet scales, which are available in many stores, have a bowl-like container that sits on the scales, which will help keep the young from falling off the scales. Record the weights. Weight gain is normally a good sign of a healthy young pet, and weight loss is a bad sign that the pet has an issue of some type. If there is no weight gain, check to make sure that the young one is getting fed. Also check for white gums; anemia can be caused by hookworms or Coccidia. If a virus gets into the litter, it is not uncommon to lose the entire litter. Keep the young warm.

Criteria	Normal Standard	Notes
Weight of:	100 grams +/- 10 grams	Double weight in:
Kittens	200–300 grams	Kittens: 2 weeks
Puppies	400–500 grams	Puppies: 10–12 days
Medium Breeds	700+ grams	
Large Breeds		
Giant Breeds		
Heart rate C & D	Above 200 beats per minute	C & D = cat and dog
Respiration C & D	15-35 <2 weeks of age	C & D = cat and dog
Body temperature	96–97° F Needs to stay close to the mother	After 1–2 weeks body temp increases. By 4 weeks body temp reaches 100° F
Jerking of limbs	Activated sleep	Prevents atrophy
Neuromuscular reflexes	Present at 7 days	
Eyes open	+/- 12–14 days	
Iris is blue–gray	Changes to adult color 4–6 weeks	
Normal vision	3–4 weeks	
Flexor Tone	Predominates first four days, causing comma body conformation of most newborns	
Extensor Tone	After four days, dominant lies on side with head extended	
Pain perception	Present at birth	
Withdraw reflexes	Not well developed until 7–14 days	
Start walking	+/- 16 days and can support own body weight	
Normal gait	+/- 21 days	

What to Look for When Doing Exams for Less Than Four-Week-Old Kittens or Puppies

Never place a kitten or puppy on a cold countertop, table, or cold metal. They will lose body heat very quickly.

- *Weight*: Check the weight with a gram scale.
- *Appearance*: Kittens or puppies should be plump and round with no gross abnormalities of size or shape.
- *Head*: The head should be mobile and exhibit rooting reflex. Feel for open spaces between the bones on the head or fontanels, or abnormal size of the head due to excess fluid production in the brain or hydrocephalus.
- *Ears*: Look for size and position.
- *Nose*: Look for fluid or other accumulations in the nostrils.
- *Mouth*: Look for harelip and cleft palate and check presence of blue or nonpink gums; the young should have a sucking reflex.
- *Skin*: Look for wounds, hydration, or dehydration and completeness of hair coat, which should be shiny and free of debris.
- *Breathing*: Breathing should be regular and unlabored. Note the rate and depth of respiration. Deep respiration may indicate a heart problem or lung infection.
- *Thorax*: Look for completeness, symmetry, wounds, rib fractures, and sterna or spinal abnormalities.
- *Abdomen*: The abdomen will be enlarged following nursing, and the puppy and kitten should be in a restful state—if restless and vocal after feeding, it is a sign that the young one may be sick or have swallowed excess air.
- *Umbilical Cord*: The cord is normally gone two to three days after birth. Make sure it is clean; it is easy to become infected, so cleanliness is important.
- *Tail, Limbs, Anus, and Genitalia*: Look to assure all are present and normal.

- *Urination and Defecation*: Both may be stimulated by rubbing the area with a moist, warm cloth. In the process, check for possible blood in the urine, loose stools, or constipation. Check the anus to assure it is present and open with no swelling or redness.

Bottle Feeding, Tube Feeding, and Avoiding Aspiration

If the mother is not available or she has dried up, it is necessary to bottle feed or to tube feed the kittens and puppies for at least the first four weeks. Homemade formulas can be made. However, it is best to use commercially available products as they normally have all the necessary nutrients and are closest to the mother's milk. The product used most by this author has been Esbilac powder and/or liquid for puppies. Pet stores have the products for bottle feeding and tube feeding. Havolac is a product for kittens and puppies. KMR liquid or powder is for kittens, and Unilact liquid or powder and Veta-Lac are for puppies and kittens.

The caloric need for most puppies and kittens is twenty-two to twenty-six Kcal per one hundred grams of body weight.

Formula Needed per 100 Grams of Body Weight

Age	Formula per 100 g body weight	Notes
1st week	13 ml per feeding 3-4 times daily	Feed less first day feedings and gradually increase feed to full amount on the 2nd or 3rd day. Feed every 2 hours
2nd week	17 ml per feeding	Feed less first day feedings and gradually increase feed to full amount on the 2nd or 3rd day. Feed every 2 hours
3rd week	20 ml per feeding	Feed less first day feedings and gradually increase feed to full amount on the 2nd or 3rd day. Feed every 3 hours

4th week	22 ml per feeding	Feed less first day feedings and gradually increase feed to full amount on the 2nd or 3rd day. Feed every 3 hours.

With a favorable response to feedings, puppies should gain one to two grams per day per pound of body weight (two to four grams per day per kilogram weight) of the anticipated adult weight for the first five months. Kittens should weigh about 80–140 grams at birth (most weigh about 100–120 grams) and gain 50–100 grams per week.

Treatment:

To bottle feed, you need to accumulate pet nursing bottles and nipples. Make sure the nipple has only one hole; you do not want to force formula into the mouth of the young. Aspiration phenomena can kill the kitten or puppy. Avoid multiple holes in the nipples as it allows too much formula into the mouth and the little one will not be able to handle the formula. If you see formula come out of the nose, you are about to do what I described. Stop what you are doing and wait. You cannot rush the young ones.

The pet nipple bottles are made especially for feeding orphaned puppies or kittens and are the preferred nipple bottle to use. Sometimes the hole in the nipple is not open as it should be. Heating a pin and sticking it into the missing nipple hole will correct the nipple problem. Be careful not to make a big hole. When feeding, place a drop of formula onto the nipple before putting it into the pet's mouth. Never squeeze milk out of the bottle while the nipple is in the animal's mouth. Doing so may result in you pumping formula directly into the lungs.

Tube feeding is the fastest way to feed a young orphan. You can do this rather easily. You need to get a feeding tube from the pet store. Use the feeding tube to measure the length that you will be putting into the orphan. Place the tube on the outside of the pet and measure on the tube from the last rib to the tip of the nose, putting a mark by the nose on the tube. Pass the tube down until the mark is at the nose—do not go further and do not go less than your measured distance.

As the orphan grows, you will need to remark the tube as it will need to go deeper as the pet ages and grows. When feeding, fill the syringe and feeding tube with warm formula, being sure to expel any air that is in the syringe or the feeding tube. Open the orphan's mouth slightly; with the animal's head held in a normal nursing position, move the tube slightly to the left to help hit the esophagus. Gently pass the tube into the pet down to the mark on the tube. If an obstruction is felt before reaching the mark, you have put the tube into the lungs. Withdraw the tube and reinsert it down to the mark on the tube. When the tube is in up to the mark, slowly press on the syringe. Over a period of two or two and a half minutes, deliver the formula into the stomach. With the tube feeding, regurgitation normally does not occur. However, if it does, remove the tube and wait until the next feeding interval.

Orphaned young should be encouraged to begin eating solid food at three or four weeks of age. Once they are eating, you can reduce the amount of formula. Weaning should not be complete until the puppy or kitten is six weeks of age or older.

Evaluating Puppies and Kittens Five Weeks to Six Months of Age

When evaluating five-week-old to six-month-old orphans, observe them at rest and at play. Check how the pet walks. Does the pet respond to strange environments? The pet should be starting on solid foods or have been on solid foods for some period.

The pet's head should appear normal, and there should be no noticeable discharges from the eyes, nose, or mouth. Teeth should be clean and look good. Gums should be pink. Some small breeds may show hydrocephalus at this time. It may be obvious—it can sometimes be unapparent or stealthy in appearance. The eyes should be adult colors; you can shine a flashlight into one eye and both pupils should become smaller.

You can check the mouth by pulling the jaw down and looking at the mouth and the throat for deep reds that would be caused by infections. You can check capillary refill time by pressing on the gums and timing the return of the pink color—it should be less than two seconds. The ears should be clean and free of mites. Ear mites often cause a black waxy substance to accumulate. Palpate the left side of the neck for swelling; megaesophagus can be found in five-week-old kittens. Affected kittens may be unable to keep food down and often vomit a lot.

Check the way the puppy walks. Does it use all four limbs or does it limp or carry a leg up? If so, there may be an associated trauma that is causing the lameness. It should have hair all over the body unless it is a hairless animal. Many parasites can cause hair loss. If the pet is a male, there should be two testicles. One or both may be intra-abdominal, which is prone to causing cancer, so a quick check is important.

Treatment:

Physical findings need to be treated. The treatment of choice depends on the condition noted. In many cases, you will be able use over-the-counter drugs, but in other cases, you will need to go to the pet's doctor. Do not overextend your personal treatment if you are not sure. Better to be on the safe side of your pet's health. After all, the reason that you complete a physical exam is to determine whether your pet is healthy or needs attention.

Death Losses of Puppies and Kittens

Death loss of kittens and puppies can be a real problem due to diseases, poor sanitation, or bacterial and viral infections. Death immediately after birth is often due to a fading puppy or kitten syndrome. It can be rather common to lose between 15 and 40 percent of a litter before they are twelve weeks of age. Of the deaths that occur in newborn animals, about half have no cause of death that can be found or noted.

We will discuss two causes of death in the young that will help reduce death loss. Hookworms and roundworms are common among the very young. Hookworms are passed in the mother's milk, creating a very early infection that drains the blood. Transplacental transfer allows roundworms to be present in the intestines after one week. Hookworms transfer through the milk from the mother cat to the kittens. It is important that the newborns receive treatment for internal parasites shortly after birth.

Treatment:

Mamma dogs may be treated to help prevent—or at least slow down—hookworm and roundworm infection due to the transplacental and mammary gland transfer of parasites. You can do this by starting daily treatment with Panacur (fenbendazole) (adult dogs should receive adult doses—see adult chart below) on day forty of pregnancy and continue for fourteen days after giving birth. The kittens and puppies should be dewormed every two weeks starting at two weeks of age and continue through sixteen weeks of age. The following chart gives the dose for both kittens and puppies based on gram weights. Do not give a young animal an adult dose—see kitten and puppy dose charts below.

Kitten and Puppy Dose of Fenbendazole
100 mg per cc Solution Available at Feed Stores

Weight	Dose in cc's (to be given by mouth)
100 grams	.1 cc
200 grams	.2 cc
300 grams	.3 cc
400 grams	.4 cc
500 grams	.5 cc
600 grams	.6 cc
700 grams	.7 cc
800 grams	.8 cc
900 grams	.9 cc
1000 grams	1 cc

See chart above for newborns.

Adult Panacur (Fenbendazole) Dose Chart

Make sure you *do not* use this dose chart for young kittens or puppies

(100 Mg/CC Panacur (Fenbendazole) Dosing Chart

(Weight times 25 divided by 100 = Dose in cc's)

Weight Pounds	Dose cc's	Weight Pounds	Dose CC's	Weight Pounds	Dose CC's	Weight Pounds	Dose CC's	Weight Pounds	Dose CC's
1	0.25	21	5.25	41	10.25	61	15.25	81	20.25
2	0.50	22	5.50	42	10.50	62	15.50	82	20.50
3	0.75	23	5.75	43	10.75	63	15.75	83	20.75
4	1.0	24	6.0	44	11.0	64	16.0	84	21.0
5	1.25	25	6.25	45	11.25	65	16.25	85	21.25
6	1.50	26	6.50	46	11.50	66	16.50	86	21.50
7	1.75	27	6.75	47	11.75	67	16.75	87	21.75
8	2.0	28	7.0	48	12.0	68	17.0	88	22.0
9	2.25	29	7.25	49	12.25	69	17.25	89	22.25
10	2.50	30	7.50	50	12.50	70	17.50	90	22.50
11	2.75	31	7.75	51	12.75	71	17.75	91	22.75
12	3.00	32	8.0	52	13.0	72	18.0	92	23.0
13	3.25	33	8.25	53	13.25	73	18.25	93	23.25
14	3.50	34	8.50	54	13.50	74	18.50	94	23.50
15	3.75	35	8.75	55	13.75	75	18.75	95	23.75
16	4.00	36	9.0	56	14.00	76	19.0	96	24.00
17	4.25	37	9.25	57	14.25	77	19.25	97	24.25
18	4.50	38	9.50	58	14.50	78	19.50	98	24.50
19	4.75	39	9.75	59	14.75	79	19.75	99	24.75
20	5.00	40	10.0	60	15.0	80	20.0	100	25.0

When Mamma Stops Cleaning Young

It is not uncommon for the mother dog to stop cleaning and taking care of the young that have just been born. This is more common in dogs—especially small breed dogs—and less frequent in cats. This phenomenon is sometimes due to the stress and tiredness due to the delivery of the young. On occasion, the mother will make no effort at all to clean the newborns. Your task is to step in and take the responsibility of cleaning the newborn puppies or kittens.

Treatment:

If you need to cut the umbilical cord, use a knife or sharp scissors. Before cutting the umbilical cord, tie the umbilical cord off approximately half-inch from the body (accuracy of distance is not important). You can use thread or dental floss to tie the umbilical cord. After tying and cutting the umbilical cord, take the kitten or puppy in both hands (with the head pointed away from you) and move the young one up and down to get the fluids out of the nose and mouth. Be careful that you do not let go or throw or drop the young one as you swing it. If the newborn is still moist, dry it off. When you are finished, move to the next one that needs your attention.

Prevention:

Make sure the mamma is healthy and free of parasites before birth. There is no assurance that this will prevent the mother from not taking care of the young; however, there is little more that you can do.

Chapter 3:
Assessing Your Pet's Health

I hear and I forget, I see and I remember. I do and I understand.

—*Confucius*

In this chapter, we will learn how to evaluate your pet's health parameters such as temperature, heart, pulse, and other health monitoring that can be done by pet owners if they just know what to do. All of these health monitoring suggestions are simple. A few require some equipment, such as a thermometer. Some of the techniques take some practice and patience as you learn how to do them and record your findings. There are several pages at the back of the book to record this data, visits to the pet's doctor, and immunizations.

Each time you complete these tasks, you will become better at doing them. Soon you will know what normal is for your pet. It is the only way you can learn what is normal for your pet so give it a go. If you have difficulty, just keep at it—you will get it down soon. Recording your findings and data is important so you can refer to what you have found in the past and compare it to new findings. For example, if heart rates, percussion sounds, or temperatures change, you will be able to compare it to your recorded normal values and know your pet has some sort of a problem. You will have the dates and times of your evaluations to compare with the dates that abnormalities were noted.

Obtaining the Temperature of Your Pet

To obtain the temperature of your pet, a rectal thermometer is the best and most accurate tool to use. Any type of rectal thermometer will be fine; if it happens to be digital, read the instructions on how to use it properly. It helps to lubricate the thermometer with a lubricant such as K-Y Jelly, Vaseline, or any other lubricant—as long as it will not cause a burning sensation.

Temperature needs to be taken when the pet is calm and not after vigorous exercise. If the pet is calm, one person will be able to obtain the temperature. Two people are a big help as you will see. When dealing with cats, it can be a bit more difficult to get the thermometer where it belongs—just be careful and do not force the thermometer. Be gentle and put slight forward pressure on the thermometer until it is in position. If it's not electronic, leave it in position for about a minute to allow the thermometer to register the temperature.

Treatment:

Normal temperatures for dog and cats range from 101^0 F (38.3^0 C) to 102^0 F (38.9^0 C), assuming the pet is in a normal temperature environment. If the conditions at the time the temperature is taken and the environment are as described, then a temperature of 103^0 F (39.4^0 C) would be a concern—and it may be an indication of a problem with your pet. However, if the pet is outside on a hot day, 103^0 F might be normal. Likewise, a low temperature below 99.5 degrees F (37.5 C) for dogs and below 100^0 F (37.8^0 C) in cats may be an indication of hypothermia. Any temperature below these should alert you to a problem. High or low temperatures may be a signal that your pet needs to be checked by your veterinarian.

Normal Respiratory Rate

I believe you can best determine what the normal rate of respiration is for your pet during any healthy period of its life. The normal range of respirations per minute is between fifteen and thirty for dogs and twenty to thirty for cats. A breath is inhalation and exhalation. Your pet has not read this book and does not know what the respiration rate is. Therefore, you need to count and establish the normal at-rest rate for your pet. Keep that number in mind over the years. If you notice a significant increase or decrease, then you can have some idea that your pet may have an issue that your veterinarian may be able to diagnose. There are so many types of respiratory issues that can be present that we will not even attempt to discuss causes of respiratory difficulty—and none are over-the-counter treatable.

Treatment:

Establish the normal respiratory rate for your pet while calm or at rest (not panting or just after exercise) to help you determine if the respiratory rate is elevated or too slow or if your pet's abdomen moves with each breath. At times, abdominal movement with every breath is an indication of difficulty breathing, which may indicate a lung infection. You now have a rough guide to help you decide if there is a need for your pet to visit the pet's doctor.

Blood Flow or Capillary Refill Time

You can get a ballpark idea of the level of blood in the body and whether it is being pumped through the body as it should be. Your pet's gums should be pink—not light pink, almost white, or white. If they are not pink, then it could be anemia. You need to determine what is causing the blood loss. Hookworms and coccidia are among the first to rule out. Secondly, you can put pressure on the gum with your finger in an area where you can see. When you apply pressure, the area under your finger—and immediately around your finger—will turn white or become blanched. Remove your finger and the white area should almost immediately return to the original pink color. If not, it can be an indication that there is less blood flowing.

Delayed blood flow might be due to a loss of blood in your pet. You can practice this on your cat or dog so you will know what it should be like and how quick the pink color of the gums returns when you put pressure on the gums with your finger. After practicing—and getting to know what the gums should look like and how fast your cat's or dog's pink color returns (capillary refill)—you will be able to identify abnormal blood flow by the capillary blood flow that you can visualize by the return of a pink color after removing pressure from the gums.

Treatment:

An easy test of blood flow is to place a finger on the pet's gums and apply pressure to cause the area under and around your finger to become white (blanch) or very light pink. Remove your finger and the pink should return within one or two seconds. This procedure is very easy to practice on your healthy pet. If you look at your pet's gums and find the gums to be pale or there is a slow return to pink after applying finger pressure to the gums (capillary refill time), then blood flow is slow. Take your pet to the pet's doctor as soon as possible.

If you cannot—or will not—take your pet to the doctor, then you can treat for hookworms and coccidia. If it is either of these parasites, the pet may be having bouts of loose stools and dehydration. If your pet is young, pale gums can be caused by panleukopenia in cats or corona virus or parvovirus in dogs. I cannot overemphasize the importance of going to the veterinarian if your pet has pale mucus membranes or slow return to pink gums. Slow return to pink, pale, or white gums normally indicates a serious disease and may be a life-or-death situation.

Obtaining Your Pet's Heart Rate

In the early days of medicine, a physician would put an ear on the chest of people and veterinarians would put an ear on the side of the chest of animals to hear the heart and lung. When the stethoscope was invented, this changed.

In years past, people did not bathe much. French physician René Theophile Hyacinthe Laennec (1781–1826) did not want to put his ear on the dirty body of a pretty, buxom young woman—and he invented the stethoscope, which was a round wooden cylinder (Sherwin B. Nuland, MD, *Doctors: The History of Scientific Medicine Revealed through Biography*, The Teaching Company, Chantilly, VA). You do not have to make your stethoscope; you can purchase one or you can put your ear to the chest of your pet to hear the heart and lungs. You can determine the heart rate in beats per minute and listen for crackling or rasping sounds within the lungs.

Treatment:

The normal heart sound you should hear is "lub dub" repeated over and over and over. Each lub dub represents one heartbeat. Normal heart rate for adult dogs is 70–160 beats per minute, toy breeds up to 180 beats per minute, puppies up to 220 beats per minute, giant breeds 60–140 beats per minute, and cats 120–240 beats per minute.

Count the beats for fifteen seconds and then multiply the beats by four to get the heart rate in beats per minute, which is how heart rate is recorded. You can put your fingers gently on the femoral artery, which runs on the inside of the thigh (approximately in the middle of the thigh). With a little practice, you will be able to find the blood vessel and feel the heartbeats due to the increase and decrease of blood pressure in the vessel.

Count the beats for fifteen seconds and multiply the number by four to obtain the heart rate. I find that one needs to listen to the heart and lungs separately. It is very difficult to listen to both at the same time to get a good feel for the conditions that are present. Further, you cannot listen to both from the same position on the chest. You will have to listen at multiple sites on the chest. Normally there are no lung sounds; lung sounds are a bad sign. Abnormal heartbeats and lung sounds may be due to disease. It is advisable to see the pet's doctor as soon as possible to rule in or rule out bad health conditions.

Tapping or Percussion

Tapping on an empty container sounds different than tapping on the same container when it has fluid in it. Thus, you can tap on the abdomen or the chest to determine if the sounds are normal or abnormal. Abnormal might signal fluid in the chest or the abdomen. You may not know what it is, but the tapping will produce a different sound if there is fluid present. You can practice this so you know what normal sounds are like; when you hear a different sound, you will know there is an issue of some type.

Treatment:

Place two or three fingers flat on the chest or abdomen. With one or two fingers on the other hand, tap on those fingers and note the sound. It should give a hollow sound. If not, there is most likely something in the chest. You can do the same with the abdomen. If you suspect abdominal fluid, place a hand on the left or right side of the abdomen. With the other, gently tap the side of abdomen on the right or left side. When you do this, the tap will produce a small wave in the fluid—and you will be able to feel the wave hit the abdominal wall on the opposite side.

If you tap different areas of a healthy dog's abdomen, you will hear different sounds—and you need to know which areas have different sounds. The sounds are different because some organs are close to the surface and give different sounds. If you get anything other than a hollow sound when you tap on the chest or abdomen—or you believe there is fluid or a solid mass in the chest—the condition is an emergency and your pet should see the doctor as soon as possible. Delays may result in the death of your pet. It is better to let the doctor determine whether it is a bad condition rather than losing your pet.

Dehydration of Dogs and Cats

Dehydration is normally a secondary health condition to some systemic disease, such as vomiting, diarrhea, kidney failure, and a host of other conditions. Dehydration can be deadly. It can be a very serious condition that needs prompt attention. This condition is best handled by your pet's favorite doctor. The main reason is to determine what is causing the dehydration.

In most cases, the underlying disease and the dehydration need to be treated simultaneously. If for some reason you cannot—or will not—take your pet to see the pet's doctor, you can attempt to treat the dehydration at home.

Treatment:

Fluids need to be given to overcome dehydration. Dehydration is calculated as a percentage of the body weight of an animal. To test for dehydration, grab a bundle of skin and pull it up. If it flops back down right away, there probably is no dehydration. Early dehydration is normally detected at +/- 5–6 percent (determined by how slow the skin raised returns to the normal position).

When skin has a slight slowness in returning the pet is about 5–6 percent dehydration. If the skin is slower at returning, then dehydration is about 7–8 percent dehydration. When the skin stays up for a little bit then goes down, it is about 9–10 percent dehydration. When the eyes of the pet are sunken into the head and the skin stays up and does not come down, it is above 10 percent and is a death omen.

As you read different references, you may find different values, but the bottom line is that the percentage is a judgment call and there is no way to be precise. Fluids can be given orally, subcutaneously (under the skin), or intravenously. Oral treatment is done by placing a dosing syringe into the mouth or by putting a feeding tube down the esophagus to the stomach and putting fluids into the stomach or forcing water down the tube. This is done by placing a syringe in the tube by the mouth and emptying the syringe via the tube into the stomach. This can be done only if the animal is not vomiting. If the pet is vomiting, this method is not effective and may require a trip to the pet's doctor.

To place a tube into the stomach, first place the tube along the side of the dog. It should extend from the tip of the nose past the last rib. With the tube on the side of the pet, place some type of mark on the tube by the nose. Placing tape around the tube at this point is easy. This mark is necessary when the tube is placed in the mouth down to the stomach; it should be at the level of the mouth when the tube is in the stomach. If the mark is far from the mouth, you may have to place the tube in the lungs. Putting fluid into the lungs is a no-no. A roll of tape can be placed in the dog's mouth and the tube passed through the center hole of the tape.

Of course, you must hold the tape in place. This makes it a lot easier to place the tube down to the stomach. These procedures are best left to your pet's doctor. There may be acid base issues associated with the dehydration, but one cannot know without the proper tests.

Chapter 4:
Developmental Abnormalities

The best proof is experience.

—*Sir Francis Bacon*

Many animals are born with no issues, but others have shortcomings of many different origins. They may be physical or unknown until they develop with time and age. Some are simple and insignificant. We have no way of knowing what they will be. Forrest Gump said, "Life is like a box of chocolates and we never know what we are going to get." Whatever it is, we have to deal with it. We can treat, prevent, or live with them, but we do what we can with what we have.

Improper Positions of Teeth (Malocclusion)

In some animals, the teeth do not come in properly due to retained baby teeth, congenital malformation of the mouth, trauma, or some other cause. Sometimes the teeth point in directions that cause trauma and pain. Some teeth may point up and cause an indentation into the roof of the mouth tissue, causing a hole in the roof of the mouth. We have seen this syndrome in several dogs. The most common is a canine tooth hitting the roof of the mouth.

Other malformations may be due to the lower jaw being too short or too long. This may cause constant saliva discharge, resulting in a reddish, moist chin or no hair on the lower chin.

Treatment:

The treatment is an issue that your veterinarian needs to attend to because a good exam may require anesthesia. For some pets, the teeth can be pulled, which will remove the tooth in the roof of the mouth syndrome or correct teeth pointing out of the mouth. Often retained baby teeth need to be removed because they can cause permanent teeth to be crooked. There is little that can be done for the short or elongated lower or upper jaw because these conditions are congenital.

Prevention:

When the dog is a puppy, look at the teeth and make sure they are normal and coming in properly. Promptly remove any retained baby teeth or teeth that are coming in crooked.

Persistent Penile Deviation

Occasionally, a male puppy will have a thin skin attachment between the prepuce and the penis. Depending on how the tissue between the prepuce and the penis is attached, when the penis is extended to urinate, it may cause the dog to spray urine on its body or a stream of urine may point in some odd direction. Most commonly, the tip of the penis is pulled down and prevents the penis from being extended from the prepuce, causing spraying on the body. The frenulum is a very thin tissue without blood vessels or nerves, but it has the strength to prevent it from breaking. As the penis is extended, it will pull the penis in odd directions.

Treatment:

Normally all that is required it to cut the thin skin or frenulum tissue with scissors or remove it from the penis and prepuce. It most commonly has little or no blood vessels or nerve innervations, so this easy procedure is normally pain-free.

Prevention:

When the puppy is born, check the penis to make sure it is normal. If there is some thin skin that causes the penis to deviate or point in an odd direction, cut the thin skin with scissors.

Corneal Deposits or Corneal Dystrophy

Corneal dystrophy is a hereditary, noninflammatory infiltration of lipids (cholesterol). The lesions are found on the cornea of either eye. There are normally no consequences of the condition other than an area of density on the cornea. To date, there is no treatment that will resolve the opacity. It will remain as long as the dog is alive.

This condition is uncommon in cats. In my career, I have not seen it in cats. On rare occasions, before testing for ulcers, I have thought corneal opacity to be corneal dystrophy. However, when I tested for corneal ulcers, it was a superficial ulcer that looked just like corneal dystrophy. This is not common, but it can be a problem to diagnose. This is why you need to have your pet's doctor examine your pet's eyes. They have the necessary tools and medicines to diagnose and treat eyes. As you know from this book, eyes can be destroyed overnight. Be wise—not sad.

Treatment:

No treatment is available for corneal lipid (corneal dystrophy). However, you need to make sure that the opacity on the cornea is in fact corneal dystrophy and not an ulcer or other pathology that would be detrimental to your pet's eyes. If there is no way you will take your pet to the pet's doctor, you can treat the eye with Terramycin, which can be obtained at feed stores. I find that many feed stores may not have the medication mentioned here, but they have another brand that can be used. Ask the feed store for help. If it is a lipid deposit, you will not hurt the pet by treating it—and if it is an ulcer, it will get well.

Prevention:

There currently is no known way to prevent accumulation of cholesterol deposits in the cornea.

Dogs Going Around and Around in Circles or Tail Chasing

A dog may turn in fast circles or alternate speeds. However, the dog will not stop going around and around. Although the dog is not focused on the tail, it is often referred to as tail-chasing. At best, this condition can be debilitating and has a potential to be life-threatening. It is known that this condition is not due to a brain lesion. It seems not to be attention-getting behavior. At times, the stimulus is the absence of the pet owner. A dog with this condition normally will not respond to commands; if interrupted, it can become aggressive. It has been suggested that the condition is obsessive-compulsive. Some obsessive-compulsive behaviors include stargazing, fly-snapping, tail-chasing, flank-sucking, and self-mutilation. They may be anxiety-based disorders. Different dogs have differences in the way they react to this syndrome. Some pets are disabled and others are somewhat disabled.

Treatment:

This condition is not treatable with any over-the-counter drugs; there is nothing an owner can provide. This discussion is provided as information for those owners who happen to have a pet with this syndrome. This condition is special and needs professional assistance. Currently there is no cure. Knowledge of this syndrome is very limited. There seem to be similarities to obsessive-compulsive disorder in humans. Some tail-chasing dogs have responded to the same types of medications as those used in humans.

In some dogs, this syndrome may be related to autism. Greater details on tail chasing is available in the April 1, 2011, Journal of the American Veterinary Medical Association, pages 883–888, if you desire more in-depth information.

Prevention:

The wide-open spaces of a farm *might* be of some help, but it is not known what causes this syndrome. More confinement leads to more tail-chasing. Attention given to the dog normally will cause the dog to stop tail-chasing. However, it usually reoccurs when the attention stops.

Ageing Process of Eye Lens (Nuclear Sclerosis to Cataracts)

Nuclear sclerosis is a normal aging process of the lens of the eye. Different animals are affected differently—and at different ages and levels of severity. You may notice a blue color starting to appear in the eye, which is an early sign of the development of nuclear sclerosis. As the process continues, the lesions in the lens become more condensed and may appear as white specks in the eye. In time, the whole lens will be involved, leading to a mature cataract. At any stage in the process, one might believe that the pet cannot see. Blindness is very easy to test for, but you need to remove the pet from familiar surroundings.

Treatment:

There is nothing you can do to prevent or stop the condition. There are some drops for this condition called OcluVet eye drops (Webster Veterinary Supply) that may be of benefit, which your pet's doctor can provide. Studies with this compound are supposed to have shown that pets with cataracts had a 79 percent reduction in opacity/density of the nuclear sclerosis. It is definitely worth trying for your pet. Unfortunately the drug is expensive—and the pet must be treated several times per day. To test for eyesight, take your pet to an unfamiliar area. Using a leash, attempt to walk the pet into objects. If the pet does not walk into walls, doors, or other objects, it sees enough to get around okay.

Prevention:

I have no way to tell you how to prevent aging. If you find out, let me know so I can stop the process myself. Be aware that there is currently no treatment for cataracts other than surgery.

Collapsing Windpipe or Trachea

Either the lack of cartilage rings or an absorption syndrome of the windpipe rings causes this condition. The rings give the windpipe structural strength. Without the rings, the windpipe collapses or flutters back and forth. When this occurs, it causes a cough reflex that makes the pet cough a lot. This can keep owners from getting sleep. To diagnose a collapsing windpipe, it is necessary to have radiographs taken. This diagnostic tool allows one to diagnose or disprove that the cough is due to a collapsing windpipe. Treatment for this condition is expensive and requires surgery to reestablish stability to the trachea. Since there are several surgical options available, your pet's doctor will need to describe them. This syndrome is most common in middle age for smaller breeds. It is rare in large breeds—and very rare in cats.

Treatment:

There is little one can do to treat collapsing windpipe. However, coughing might be aided by Robitussin-DM. Give 2 cc or ½ teaspoon to a small dog and 5 cc or one teaspoon to a larger dog.

The Aged Cat and Dog (Geriatric Pet)

I was asked to add this subject and will attempt to put it into perspective for you. All things on the planet age—and pets are, unfortunately, no exception. With age, systems of the body tend to slow down and lose functionality. When this occurs, we call this process geriatric or aged. In reality, the same slowdown and loss of function can—and does—occur throughout life. It is usually more pronounced during the later stages of life.

I have had old cats and dogs that are as healthy and active as a puppy or kitten. We tend to think of advanced age as a failure of systems, such as thyroid dysfunction, intestinal issues, bone issues, urinary issues, and others. The systems become unglued with age—this is life. A book can be written on each of these subjects. None of us has a crystal ball to allow us to know what will or will not occur. Frequently there is little an owner can do to diagnose these issues—and often not much one can do to treat the condition without the aid of the pet's doctor.

We will divide aged into early-, middle-, and late-aged. The early-aged is a time in the pet's life when systems start to slow down. Perhaps they are not as fast on the run—and less inclined to do so—but they still do. At times, they are just like the old days, outrunning you or playing with a ball like a puppy. Conditions of multiple systems are just starting to go, but they are not what they once were.

Middle-aged systems are a bit more on the blitz and may cause more trips to the doctor for pain medication or treatment, but the pet is still doing pretty well. In late-age, our emotions start to kick in. We love the pet and hate to see the conditions that have developed. Perhaps the pet urinates on the floor, does not make it to the litter box, or does not want to go outside. We know the end is approaching, but we are going to have to make that fateful decision sooner or later. It often boils down to what we are willing to tolerate with the old gal or guy. It is tough decision time.

Treatment:

Certainly there are treatments that the aged pet can endure for its ailments. However, most conditions of the aged pet are extensive and involve an organ system. The older pet health issues are normally complex, require special medicines, and need special careful handling to make sure the pet can endure the necessary treatment that will allow the condition to be healed and have a healthy, happy conclusion. This, of course, is not always possible.

Health conditions for the aging often progress to an end point beyond which there is very limited medical aid that can improve the condition. Cancer, neurological deficits, poor lung health, heart issues, and a multitude of other conditions almost always require money and your pet's doctor to help to make the pet's life palatable. Unfortunately, there is often not a cure—only palatable end points of the acquired disease or condition. On the other hand, just because the pet is aged, there should be no hesitations to aid the pet for its health conditions.

Focus on the condition—not the age—when making decisions. If a pet has a heart condition and needs surgery, it may be untreatable. The heart condition may have developed as a progressive disease that the dog has lived with for a period of time. On the other hand, if the pet has two subcutaneous tumors the size of a softball—and the other systems are good—then it is a go. If a health condition, even with treatment, is a short-term life extension, then one has to factor in quality of life. Is it the right thing to do? It is a tough decision—and you know that you have to do what you have to do. No one else can do so.

Euthanasia

Euthanasia is most often defined as an easy or painless death. Unfortunately, many of us have had to face this with our pets. There are many causes for the need to euthanize a pet. The good news is that there are humane ways to end suffering for pets. The bad news is that tough decisions have to be made—and extreme emotions accompany those decisions. There is no easy way to let go of a pet you love, but you have to do what you have to do. There is no such thing as an easy way out—you have to make the decision. In my career, I could tell sad story after sad story. Even after many years, many cases bring tears to my eyes—and they were not my pets. We understand—and we do what we can to ease the trauma of euthanasia.

Treatment:

In my humble opinion, the most humane method is with drugs available to a veterinarian. The American Veterinary Medicine

Association has an online website http://www.avma.org/issues/animal_welfare/euthanasia.pdf that describes many approved methods of euthanasia that are considered to be humane ways to euthanize an animal. In our community, one can take the pet to the Orange County Animal Services and turn in the animal for euthanasia—and it is probably the least expensive way to complete the task. Many communities have this option, but the best way is to take the pet to your pet's favorite doctor.

Prevention:

Unfortunately, some try to euthanize their pet using nonacceptable methods. I believe strongly that euthanasia should be performed humanely by professionals who have been trained to complete these procedures. There have been newspaper articles about folks attempting to euthanize their pets that were unsuccessful and caused severe pain. Euthanasia is stressful enough without causing pain and unusual sounds from your pet. Having your pet taken care of by the pet's doctor will assure you that the procedure is completed humanely.

How Will I Know When to Euthanize?

This is a very personal decision. The most common reasons for euthanasia are quality of life, extreme trauma or pain, and terminal illnesses. Many folks do not have the financial means to pay for expensive veterinary medical bills associated with certain diseases and trauma.

I recall a cat that somehow fell into an electric transformer station. When it came to the clinic, it smelled cooked and looked absolutely horrible. That animal was euthanized. My pen pal in San Antonio had a Doberman that was diagnosed with cancer. He wrote to ask my opinion. I suggested euthanasia, but he opted for treatment. Several thousand dollars later, he had the pet euthanized. He wrote me several times later saying he should have listened, but it was not my decision.

One lady asked about a brain tumor in her ten-year-old dog. He was having seizures, chronic pain, and blindness. She had already made up her mind, but she needed my support. I had another case in which the dog's body had turned to stone and the cords to the heart valves had broken. Its lungs were filling with fluid extremely fast, but the person could not say the words. He cried and cried before slobbering out the words.

Everyone wants to be sure that they are doing the right thing because it is so difficult to let go. I could probably write a book on all the different scenarios that I have dealt with over the many years, but the bottom line was quality of life, pain, and terminal diseases.

Treatment:

The best options are personal. The owner of the pet must make the tough decision that no one else can make for you. When a person discusses options with me, they totally want assurance that they are making the correct decision for their beloved pet. They need to talk to a person that they trust and put faith in. It is tough to keep from becoming emotional with the person making the decision. The emotions can be so thick that one can cut them with a knife. We fully understand your anguish, but you must do what you have to do. Often when coping with these procedures, one feels remorse or that they could have done more. Their feelings are normal and experienced by many. Do not feel ashamed to feel remorse and deep loss—it is one of the greatest losses you experience.

If you need further help dealing with the loss of your pet, the following pet loss support and grief counseling websites provide more great information and telephone numbers to help you through the process. To find the information, look for the pet loss support on the site. I found that putting "pet loss" or "pet loss grieving" in the website search normally would bring up the information being looked for.

Pet Loss Support and Grief Counseling Centers

Chicago VMA 630-325-1600
www.chicagovma.org

Colorado State University, Argus Institute: 970-297-124
www.argusinstitute.colostate.edu

Cornell University: 607-253-3932
www.vet.cornell.edu

University of Illinois: 217-244-2273 or 877-394-2273
vetmed.illinois.edu

Michigan State University: 517-432-2696
Cvm.msu.edu

The Ohio State University: 614-292-1823
Vet.osu.edu

Tufts University:
www.tufts.edu/vet

Virginia Tech/University of Maryland: 540-231-8038
www.vetmed.vt.edu

Washington State University: 509-335-5704 or 866-266-8635
www.vetmed.wsu.edu

Unexpected Reactions to Drugs in Cats and Dogs

There is always a potential that any drug or compound might cause
an unexpected reaction. There is no way to know if the pet will have
a reaction to any compound—including food—until it happens.
Of course, once you know that your pet will respond to a particular

drug, compound, or food, whatever caused the reaction cannot be given again. Some of the most common acute reactions include vomiting, anorexia, depression, lethargy, loose stools or diarrhea, convulsions, and trembling.

How frequently do adverse drug reactions occur? It is impossible to know the number of adverse reactions. I have seen adverse reactions due to immunizations, but not to any specific immunization. The bad news is that even a pet that has had no issues in the past can have an adverse reaction. Hair loss, skin rashes, and eye infections are a few reactions than can occur.

Treatment:

The best thing that you can do for most immunization reactions is to give a dose of Benadryl to your pet (see the dose chart in Chapter 1). The cause and type of reaction will dictate the most appropriate treatment. For some compound reactions, simply stopping the compound will result in resolution; others may need the help of the pet's doctor. If it is an immunization reaction, the pet should respond to the Benadryl within thirty minutes. If it is not resolved in that time, you may need to take your pet to see the pet's doctor. Limited experience or the inability to control emotions or recognize bad reactions result in the need for extensive treatments. Treatments may include starting your pet on intravenous drips, holding the animal for prolonged period of time, and treating for other signs.

Severe reactions can result in death. Be alert to the reactions and be proactive in getting the pet treated either by yourself or the pet's doctor.

Prevention:

Immediately eliminate the drug, compound, or food that is responsible for the reaction. Do not reuse any of the compounds. Watch for the first reaction because there is no way to know if a pet will have a bad reaction to any compound or food until it happens.

Contact Skin Problems or Hives

Hives are not common in dogs or cats, but they do occur. Hives are caused by the pet coming into contact with plants, compounds, or other irritants. Terrier breeds, French Poodles, and golden retrievers are most commonly affected, but that does not preclude others from having this syndrome. The signs are observable and most often are skin reactions. You may see patchy areas of skin swelling or skin discoloration that is red. This condition comes on rapidly and can involve respiratory aspects that cause difficulty in breathing. Normally signs are in direct relation with the length of time in contact with the substance—and how sensitive the pet is to hive-producing compounds or plants.

Treatment:

If you happen to see early signs of hives, remove the pet from the area. Removing the pet from the environment will reduce exposure—and help reduce the reaction. Furthermore, if you remove the pet from the area, you will have time on your side. The hives will resolve without treatment if the stimulus of the hives is not present. However, treatment will certainly hasten the resolution of the hives.

Benadryl in pill or liquid form can be purchased at Wal-Mart, pharmacies, and grocery stores. Dosage charts can be found in Chapter 1. If you think the substance can be washed off, give the pet a bath. It may be necessary to visit your pet's doctor to get better—and perhaps faster-reacting—drugs. Hives can result in serious respiratory dysfunction. If need be, seek professional help and necessary drugs. Your pet's doctor will know what to do.

Prevention:

If you know the cause of the hives, keep the pet away from the plants or offending compounds. It is often impossible to know what the stimulus to the allergy is.

Collie Breed Seizures due to Ivermectin

Certain breeds of dogs cannot tolerate treatment with Ivermectin. Ivermectin is used to treat skin parasites, treat internal parasites, and treat or prevent heartworms. Collies and related breeds can transport Ivermectin into the brain and spinal column (central nervous system). Once it is in, it cannot get out. Your pet might experience violent seizures or die. This syndrome is related to the gene currently referred to as the mutant ABCB1-1Δ (formerly the MDR1 gene).

The gene has been studied in France and Australia; it has the same percentage of inheritance for dogs in the United States. The percentage of affected dogs runs about 35 percent that are affected with the mutant ABCB1-1Δ and will most likely react to Ivermectin, 45 percent are carriers and may or may not respond to Ivermectin, and 20 percent are not affected and can be treated with Ivermectin.

The College of Veterinary Medicine at Washington State University has done extensive studies. Affected breeds include Australian shepherd, Australian shepherd Mini, Border Collies, Collies, English Shepherds, German Shepherds, Herding Breed Cross, Long-haired Whippets, McNab, Silken Windhounds, mixed breeds, and Shetland Sheepdogs.

You can find charts at http://www.vetmed.wsu.edu/depts-VCPL/breeds.aspx and at http://www.mwcr.org/be_aware.htm.

Treatment:

Currently there are not many options that are available for treatment of these breeds. In the future, new drugs may become available that can be used in these breeds. Check with your pet's doctor about to the availability of such drugs for use in your collie breed dogs. Other than to do all you can to keep your pet from being bitten by heartworm-transmitting mosquitoes, there is not much more you can do. Currently, no over-the-counter drug can be safely used for the listed breeds. Your favorite veterinarian will be able to advise you on what to do to protect your pet. The only way to know if your dog has the mutant gene is to have your dog tested.

Prevention:

The College of Veterinary Medicine at Washington State University has a test kit that is free and easy to perform. The test will let you know if your pet has ABCB1-1Δ. The Veterinary College will send instructions on how to collect the sample and will explain the results to you. You can order a test kit online at http://www.mwcr.org/be_awre.htm. Click on the "Order a Test Kit Online." Or go to http://www.vetmed.wsu.edu/depts-VCPL/test.aspx and click on "Test Your Dog" and "Instructions for Pet Owners." Contact the university at 509-335-3745, VCPL@vetmed.wsu.edu, or Veterinary Clinical Pharmacology Lab, P.O. Box 609, Pullman, WA 99163-0609. Or you can take your dog to see your favorite veterinarian.

Chapter 5:
Diseases

Energy and persistence conquer all things.
—*Benjamin Franklin*

Disease has been around from the start of time and continues today. We are learning how to overcome some, but others remain a mystery. As we meet with issues, we need to roll up our sleeves and tackle them. In this chapter, we look at conditions, provide a treatment or a means to have it treated, and suggest how the condition can be prevented.

Coonhound Paralysis

This condition is common in dogs but rare in cats. Signs of this disease normally begin to show seven to fourteen days after a dog has been bitten or scratched by a raccoon. The cause is not completely known, but it is believed that it is an immune reaction to raccoon saliva. The dog will become flaccid and will be unable to walk or get up. The dog is normally able to eat—and urination, defecation, and tail movement are present. The dog will need to be fed and require special care. In severe cases, the dog may die from respiratory failure. The dog normally continues to be able to perceive or feel pain if a pain stimulus is applied. Some dogs and cats can have this syndrome without coming in contact with a raccoon. This is known as idiopathic paralysis—and no cause is currently known. However, signs and treatment are the same.

Treatment:

Treatment is constant care, cleaning, feeding, and providing soft bedding so the dog does not develop pressure skin sores or ulcers. In most cases, the pet will recover or improve within two weeks, but complete recovery can take up to six months. If the response to the coonhound paralysis is severe, the muscles will seem to become smaller or disappear. The pet might never completely recover from the muscle loss or so called muscle atrophy. Relapse can reoccur if the dog is bitten again by a raccoon.

Prevention:

This syndrome is prevented by ensuring that your pet is not bitten by a raccoon. There is no prevention for idiopathic paralysis.

Warts or Papilloma of the Mouth and Skin

There seems to be nothing that is simple and straightforward—and oral warts are no exception. There is more than one syndrome for this disease. However, this discussion will focus on those warts affecting younger dogs (six months to four years of age). It attacks the skin (mucus membranes) on the inside of the mouth and lips. Warts in the esophagus can cause difficulty swallowing.

Warts are benign little tumors that are caused by viruses. Skin warts are more often seen in males. It has been put forward that the aggressive interactivity of males may be the reason for this. It is contagious for other dogs through contact—but not for the owners. Depending upon the location, size, and numbers of warts in the mouth, the growths can get in the way of chewing or swallowing. They can also result in excessive drooling, oral discomfort, and bad breath.

Treatment:

Even though there is a wart vaccine that has been used with some success, treatment can be frustrating. Warts are somewhat self-limiting. Warts can take a long time to heal. It is not uncommon for them to go away in one or two months. I have scraped some warts on the lips until I made the area beneath the wart bleed. The warts seemed to go away sooner.

In people, planter warts are on the superficial or upper layer of the skin (epidermis) or the area where there are no blood vessels. Because there are no blood vessels in this area, the immune system cannot be stimulated and the pet's body is unable to respond to the infection. If the virus gets into the area under the superficial layer of the skin, the immune system is stimulated to respond—and the warts will resolve quicker. It is reasonable to believe that the same thing happens in animal warts. Your veterinarian is best qualified and prepared to help you treat this condition. Warts look unsightly and gross—people may think you are mistreating your pet—so consider having the pet's doctor handle this condition for you.

Prevention:

Wart vaccines have not been overly successful—in most cases they have had disappointing results—but they are available. However, if you are having wart problems, I would recommend getting your pets vaccinated for warts.

Drooling of Cats and Dogs (Ptyalism)

Drooling (ptyalism) is not common in cats or dogs. Its presence most often indicates a transient excitement neuro-stimulation, being transported in a car, the presence of a bad tooth, a foreign body in the mouth, throat region of the animal, a blockage, objects under the tongue, inability to swallow, or a system disease. We will focus on the excitement neuro-stimulation and not the disease process of drooling.

Cats and dogs have been noted to produce excessive saliva when taken in a car. This is probably due to the excitement of the environment that the animal is not accustomed to. The excitement causes a neurological response, producing more saliva than usual. The excitement or motion of a vehicle stimulates this response while being transported or shortly after arrival. Also a new environment can stimulate this response.

Normally this is not a disease. This can be determined by the fact that it started in the car or shortly after arrival. I have seen this occur in cats—particularly on the day after travel and being placed in a new environment. My daughter took her nineteen-year-old cat to the veterinary clinic because it had been drooling for a day. A bad tooth was causing the drooling and keeping the cat from eating. When the doctor pulled the tooth, the cat began eating and the drooling stopped.

It only takes seconds to check the mouth, throat, and under the tongue. Watch the pet and allow a few minutes after the pet gets accustomed to its new environment—nonpathogenic drooling will usually be resolved. If it is persistent, your pet needs to see the doctor.

Treatment:

Normally there is no treatment necessary for momentary or transportation-stimulated drooling. Be patient and give the animal some time. Usually it will subside and resolve itself unless there is underlying pathology. A quick check of the throat, mouth, and under the tongue for foreign bodies is very easy. A little pressure on the teeth might show a need for removing a tooth.

Prevention:

There is no preventing travel drooling, but Benadryl has been used effectively in some pets. If your pet tends to drool in the car, Benadryl about twenty to thirty minutes before travel helps. Benadryl is not always effective, but it is worth a try and may be effective. A Benadryl dosage chart can be found in Chapter 1. Start with a low does and increase dosage as needed.

Eating Garbage or Food Poisoning

This condition is most often seen in dogs. Cats tend to be finicky eaters, but dogs tend to wolf everything down. If you have experienced bad food, you know how your dog feels. The signs in the dog are very close to those seen in people. Signs of food poisoning include vomiting, loose stools, lethargy, no interest in eating, and a reluctance to move.

Treatment:

If you see the dog consume spoiled food, you can use hydrogen peroxide to induce vomiting. However, most often the activity is not observed. If the dog vomited the spoiled food, it is less of a concern. The issue is how much the dog consumed and how much has been vomited. Your veterinarian can supplement treatment with drugs that stimulate vomiting (emetics) or other medications. Other medications or treatments can flush the intestinal tract if necessary. A warm water enema until the dog vomits is simple (through and through enema)—but very messy.

Prevention:

Keep your pet away from garbage. The more decomposed the garbage is, the worse it is for your pet.

Lead Poisoning in Pets

One cause of lead poisoning is being shot by a shotgun. If the pet lives, it is not poisonous; the pet will be fine even with the lead shot in its body. The other cause is consumption or getting the lead into the intestinal tract so that it can be absorbed into the body like other nutrients.

Lead poisoning is not as common as it used to be, but there are still sources of lead that can be very harmful to your pet. The most common is lead-based paint. Modern paints are not lead-based. However, if you happen to live in an older home, there is a considerable chance that the house has lead-based paint. Other sources for lead poisoning include batteries, golf balls, roofing materials, curtain weights, fishing sinkers, lead pellets and shot, and lead pipes. The syndrome is more prevalent in younger pets. Cats of all ages also tend to chew on different things.

Signs of lead poisoning or toxicity depend on the dosage. Acute lead poisoning is due to a large intake of lead; chronic lead poisoning is due to repeated doses. Acute signs include lethargy, not eating, abnormal behavior, tremors, seizures, and blindness. Signs of chronic lead poisoning are obscure and may not be noticeable. Advance poisoning includes lethargy, not eating, not doing well, vomiting, diarrhea, abnormal behavior, seizures, and pale (or bluish) mucus membranes.

Treatment:

Prevention is the best option. Prevent the pet from getting any lead-containing items. The most common is paint in older homes or batteries. Once the pet is poisoned, your pet must see the doctor as the treatment can be rather involved and prolonged, depending on the severity of the toxicity. Lead toxicity requires blood testing to determine its cause and requires prescription drugs to treat the condition, which can be expensive.

Prevention:

It definitely pays to keep items containing lead away from your pets. If you have items that contain lead, store these items away from your pets. This will pay big dividends and keep pet healthy—and pet medical bills costs low. I personally have seen this syndrome more often in cattle than small animals due to farmers throwing old car batteries out in a pasture where cows lick them. Small animals will also lick old batteries.

Identifying Flea Allergy Dermatitis on Your Pet

It is very common for dogs and cats to have flea allergy dermatitis if the pet is not being treated routinely for fleas. Too often, folks treat their pet only once or twice a year—and sometimes never. The most classic signs appear after a prolonged period of nontreatment for fleas. The pet will start to lose hair or have a thinning of hair on the lower back in the lumbar area (just in front of the tail). The longer the pet is not treated, the worse the hair loss becomes. With advanced flea allergy dermatitis, the hair loss starts to move up the back toward the head. There can be hair loss down the back legs as well. You may notice your pet biting a lot in the lumbar region. *How to Treat Your Dogs and Cats with Over-the-Counter Drugs* discussed finding of granules on the skin of cats, which is military eczema or dermatitis and a sign of lots of fleas on your pet.

Normally a pet biting in the region of the tail is due to fleas being present on the back or flea allergy dermatitis, which will respond to the bite of only one flea at any location on the body. The flea bite will cause of the pet to scratch or bite the area.

Treatment:

Treatment is simple. All you have to do is treat for fleas. However, if your pet has hair loss, it will take several months of treatment to get the hair to grow back. The hair loss occurs over a period of time—and it will take time to get the hair to grow back . Be consistent and persistent with your treatment and the hair will grow back in time. I recommend Advantage II for cats and Advantix II for dogs. These medicines are available online or at PetSmart and Petco. They are also found in some military PX or BX facilities. Advantage II and Advantix II kills fleas, flea larvae, and flea eggs. These simple new products work very well. Your pet will appreciate it—and will look much better with hair than without hair.

Prevention:

Treat for fleas every month. Put the product on the skin on the back of the neck.

Back-and-Forth Movement of the Eye (Nystagmus)

Back-and-forth movement of the eye is not normal in animals. The movement normally will have what is known as a fast and a slow component. In other words, as the eye moves in one direction, the movement will be fast and the other direction slower than the fast movement. The movement of the eye is repetitive, rapid, and involuntary. The eye can move horizontally, in a rotary motion, or vertically.

The three types of nystagmus are vestibular, idiopathic vestibular, and pendular.

Vestibular nystagmus (semicircular canals of the ear) is the movement of the eye. It is normally horizontal, but it can be rotary—or even vertical—with a fast and slow segment of the eye movement. The fast movement is away from the side of the ear infection (vestibular infection semicircular canals), and the slow movement is in the direction of the ear infection (vestibular infection semicircular canals). Vestibular nystagmus may be associated with vomiting, difficulty walking or not being able to walk, circling, body rolling, and head tilt. This is most often due to a chronic ear infection that has been ignored by the owner. As the ear is treated, the eye movements may correct as the ear heals. Given time—and if the ear is cleared up—the nystagmus normally will resolve.

Idiopathic vestibular nystagmus is due to a central lesion in the brain and tumors, infections, or trauma. The lesion determines whether the condition can be treated. Due to the lesion, facial or cranial nerve involvement may cause facial paralysis.

Pendular nystagmus has no fast or slow movement. It is back and forth—and is the most uncommon of the three types. This type of nystagmus is congenital. There is no progression of the nystagmus; the chief complaint is normally limited eye movements.

Treatment:

Vestibular nystagmus is prevented by keeping the pet's ears clean. If the owner has failed to keep the ears clean and the pet develops nystagmus, then diagnosis of the type of nystagmus and the medication needed will be determined by the pet's doctor. Unknown origin nystagmus or idiopathic may not be treatable, but your veterinarian will have to determine if it is a central brain lesion and what can be done. Pendular nystagmus is not treatable.

Prevention:

Of the three kinds of nystagmus, only vestibular nystagmus can be prevented by keeping ears clean and clear of ear mites. A technique for cleaning ears can be found in Chapter 1 in *How to Treat Your Dogs and Cats with Over-the-Counter Drugs*. There is no way to predict if an animal will get brain tumors. If you are a Civil War buff, it might be of interest to know that Mrs. Ulysses S. Grant had nystagmus—and always turned her head when being photographed. The right side of her head is shown in almost every photograph.

Cats Are Better Than Dogs at Hiding Illness

Behavioral changes can be early signs of illness in pets. These changes are often less obvious in cats than in dogs. Cat owners may not notice subtle changes in appetite, bowel habits, or behavior until an illness or condition is rather advanced. Cats age much faster than people; their major health changes can occur in short periods of time. With increasing age, the risk of cancer, periodontal disease, obesity, kidney disease, thyroid disease, and diabetes increases.

Treatment:

The best way to unmask hidden insidious disease is to take your pet to the pet's doctor on a routine basis. By doing this simple task, you will unmask hidden illness early in the disease process—and help catch the condition early so it can be treated. Wellness plans have proven to extend lives of pets considerably. Due to a cat's increasing age and the possibilities of cats obtaining many systemic diseases, I recommend that your cat visit the cat's doctor a minimum of two times per year.

The justification for such visits it to catch nonrecognizable disease processes early so that they can be treated and overcome before the disease advances and it is too late or treatment is too extensive and expensive. Good health care will extend the life of your pet considerably.

If you shudder at the expense, just save a few coins between visits so when the time comes you will have the means to do so—you will be so glad you did.

Prevention:

Wellness plans are prevention plans. They save money and add many happy years to the life of your pet. It might cost a little more, but your pet depends on you.

After Birth Tremors of Mamma Dogs and Cats

Post-delivery of young puppies or kittens can result in tremors for dogs and cats—and the condition can progress to convulsions. This syndrome normally occurs within forty days of delivery but more commonly within the first three weeks. This condition is much more common in small breeds of dogs that have large litters than in cats.

Any size of dog may experience post-parturition tremors. Although rare, it can occur during late gestation. This condition is most often referred to as eclampsia. If any of you have personally experienced eclampsia, rest assured that the dog and cat eclampsia is not at all like the syndrome of people.

The tremors are due to the lack of calcium in the mother's blood. One of the major causes is inappropriate supplementation of calcium during pregnancy. One would think that supplementation of calcium would be the right thing to do, but it turns out to be a cause of the syndrome—and actually makes the disease more likely to occur. Furthermore, the calcium supplementation upsets the calcium balance of the mother and prevents the balanced absorption of food calcium. Calcium should *never* be given to the mother during pregnancy due to the disruption of the normal balance of calcium in the body. An alert owner may notice signs in the mother before the tremors begin, including panting, restlessness, mild tremors, twitching, muscle spasms, and gait changes (stiffness and ataxia). There can be behavior changes as well as aggression, whining, salivation, and pacing.

Another cause is feeding foods that have inappropriate calcium-phosphorus ratios, such as all-meat diets. People often feed small dogs too much striated muscle, causing a big problem in dog calcium levels. The drain of calcium for the formation of the puppies and the milk consumed by the puppies can be the major cause of the loss of the mother's calcium levels. This syndrome can be a life-threatening condition for your female pet. It is important to do what is right to prevent the disease.

Treatment:

Like so many diseases, prevention is the goal to strive for. You can do so by feeding a good balanced ratio to your female dog. If the dog or cat develops tremors, the condition is out of your hands. Your dog needs the help of your pet's doctor as this is a life-or-death issue. Sometimes after the doctor treats mamma dog, the calcium levels will not allow the puppies to continue to feed on the mother's milk. You may be directed by the veterinarian to hand-feed the puppies for a few days. If the mamma dog's appetite decreases, and you cannot hand-feed the puppies—or are unable to give the medications prescribed by the doctor—you may need the doctor to lend a hand. It is important that the dog remain healthy during pregnancy and post-partum periods.

Sago Palm Is the Kiss of Death for Dogs and Cats

I had no intention of discussing this topic. However, my neighbor's daughter's dog ate some sago palm and became extremely sick. The veterinarian thought the dog was going to die because its liver enzymes were off the charts. The doctor did a lot of research and found that the best treatments are over-the-counter products. My neighbor was extremely interested in the cause of the liver damage and wanted me to be sure to tell you how to treat your pets if they eat sago palm—and any other liver damage that might occur from other causes or toxins.

In all cases, it will take your pet's doctor to make the diagnosis of liver damage. My neighbor's daughter's dog is doing very well after treatment with over-the-counter products. The extent of the toxicity that any pet will experience is directly attributed to the part of the plant consumed (seeds are most toxic), the amount consumed, and the potency of the poison. The seeds, fruit, and base have heavy concentrations of cycasin, a toxin that causes liver failure within hours or days. The extent of the damage to the liver depends on the amount eaten.

The products for treatment are available online and can be purchased at most vitamin stores, pharmacies, and some grocery stores that carry vitamins. You do not have time to wait for the mail to deliver the product.

Treatment:

The best treatment is prevention. Remove the plant from your home or place it in an area where your pets cannot get to it. If you keep the plant where your pet can get to it—and you see your pet consume a part of the plant—induce vomiting as soon as possible to prevent any absorption of the toxin. Since the toxins work fast, quick action is necessary to save your pet. For dogs, vomiting can be induced by your veterinarian or by using hydrogen peroxide. Mixing equal amounts of milk and hydrogen peroxide helps the medicine go down. It is not recommended for use in cats. If you have ipecac, give dogs .5 cc to 1 cc per pound of body weight up to a maximum of 15 cc's in large dogs. The dose for cats is 1–6 cc's by mouth. A concentrated salt solution can be made quickly by heating water and adding salt. When it cools, the salt will settle. The salt water is a good for inducing vomit.

Since dogs and cats do not love these products, you must force them down. It is important that the product reaches the stomach. When you induce vomiting, you should be outside. It is common for the owner to find some sago palm in the vomit. It may be too late to induce vomiting, but the pet's doctor may be able to give a good enema to remove any sago palm that has gotten into the gut.

The following dosage chart for SAM-e and milk thistle can be followed to treat liver damage caused by sago palm. It may be necessary to cut tablets in half or quarters to get close to recommended doses. The products do not have any toxic issues. Both have been given at higher dosages without any noted issues.

The length of the treatment period is normally determined by the resolution of high liver damage enzymes. A blood chemistry test will determine the effectiveness of the treatment. However, if you do not have blood work done, the pet should respond pretty well after two weeks of treatment with SAM-e and milk thistle. If the pet is responding well, then one additional week of treatment should be completed. If there is no response after two weeks, the prognosis is very poor. Both SAM-e and milk thistle can be purchased at The Vitamin Shoppe and GNC. These stores tend to have multiple dose tablets and capsules available.

In the charts below the dosing of SAM-e and milk thistle is based on the size of the tablet or capsule and exact mg dose is impossible. You cannot get the exact dose by splinting either tablets or capsules. Also you may not be able to find the exact mg size tablets or capsules at your vitamin store. Use a tablet or capsule that is close to the indicated dose in the following charts. Much larger doses of SAM-e and milk thistle have been given without side effects.

Special note: no dose has been set by the FDA as they consider these drugs to be nutritional supplements

SAM-e (S-Adenosyl-Methionine)
Daily Dose Chart Sam-E Dose for Dogs and Cats

Weight in Pounds	Number of 90 Mg Tablets	Weight in Pounds	Number of 225 or 200 Mg Tablets
1–12	1	35–65	2
12–25	2	65–90	3
		Over 90 Pounds	4

Daily dose of SAM-e can be calculated based on 8.6 mg/pound or 18 mg/kg weight (round to the closest tablet size or combination of sizes)

(Plumb's Veterinary Drug Handbook, Sixth Edition, p. 1088–1087

Milk Thistle (Silymarin {sil-e-mar-in}) Low Dose for Dogs*

WEIGHT IN POUNDS	NUMBER OF 70 MG CAPSULES	NUMBER OF 125 MG CAPSULES	NUMBER OF 250 MG CAPSULES	NUMBER OF 300 MG CAPSULES	MG GIVEN BY THIS DOSE	NUMBER OF CAPSULES GIVEN
5-7	1				70	1
8-12		1			125	1
13-25			1		250	1
26-30				1	300	1
31-35	1			1	370	2
36-40		1		1	425	2
41-45	2			1	440	3
46-55			1	1	550	2
56-65				2	600	2
66-75		1		2	725	3
76-85			1	2	850	3
86-94				3	900	3
96-100		1		3	1025	4

*Ideal dose is 10 mg per pound every 12 hours
Milligrams column is given due to unknown availability of sizes of capsules in your communities
Plumb's Veterinary Drug Handbook 6th edition p1101-1103

Milk Thistle (Silymarin {sil-e-mar-in}) High Dose for Dogs**

WEIGHT IN POUND	NUMBER OF 70 MG CAPSULES	NUMBER OF 125 MG CAPSULES	NUMBER OF 250 MG CAPSULES	NUMBER OF 300 MG CAPSULRS	MG GIVEN BY THIS DOSE	NUMBER OF CAPSULES GIVEN
5-7	1	1			195	2
13-25	1			2	670	3
26-30		1		2	725	3
31-35			2	2	850	4
36-40		1		3	1025	4
41-45			1	3	1150	4
46-55	1	1		4	1395	6
56-65		1		5	1625	6
66-75				6	1870	7
76-85				7	2100	7
86-94			1	7	2350	8
96-100		1		8	2525	9

**Ideal dose is 25 mg per pound every 12 hours

Milligrams column is given due to unknown availability of sizes of capsules in your communities

Milk Thistle (Silymarin {sil-e-mar-in}) Low Dose for Cats***

WEIGHT IN POUNDS	NUMBER OF 70 MG CAPSULES	MG GIVEN BY THIS DOSE	NUMBER OF CAPSULES GIVEN
5-10	1/8	8.75	1/4
11-20	1/4	17.5	1/2
21-25	1	70	1

***Low dose chart ideal dose is 2 mg per pound every 12 hours

Milk Thistle (Silymarin {sil-e-mar-in}) High Dose for Cats ****

WEIGHT IN POUND	NUMBER OF 70 MG CAPSULES	MG GIVEN BY THIS DOSE	NUMBER OF CAPSULES GIVEN
5-10	1/2	35	1/2
11-20	1	70	1
21-25	1 1/4	87.5	11/4

****High dose chart ideal dose is 4 mg per pound every 12 hours
Remember splitting tables or cutting capsules is only ball park
accuracy for dose

Prevention:

The prevention for sago palm is to not to have any around if you
have pets or to keep it in area where your pet cannot get to any part
of the plant. Even old or dead parts of the plant are toxic.

Incidence of Rabies in Dogs and Cats

The good news is that the number of rabies cases reported in dogs
and cats is down. The bad news is that the majority of rabies cases
have been in cats. Therefore, cats represent 62 percent of all rabies
in all domestic pets. Cats are less likely to have been immunized
for rabies than any other domestic animal. The number of rabies
cases tends to be higher where there are raccoons. Raccoons are a
major source of rabies infections for pets. (*JAVMA*, Sept. 15, 2011,
p. 773–783)

Raccoons visiting neighborhoods at night are also a major source
of flea contamination in shaded areas. Treating sunny areas has
proven not to be of any benefit because the fleas are in shaded
areas.

Treatment:

The treatment is very simple. Make sure your pets are immunized for
rabies. Most states have laws that require rabies immunizations for
pets by the age of sixteen weeks. Normally the first immunization is

good for one year, but subsequent immunizations are good for three years. You might be aware that adjuvanted, three-year rabies vaccines can and have caused malignant tumors (sarcomas). These tumors have been reported in dogs, cats, ferrets, and horses. Alternatives to adjuvanted vaccine products are available.

Prevention:

Obtain rabies immunizations for your pets. It is better to have a protected pet. Unfortunately, many folks believe that if their pet is in the house all the time, it does not need immunizations. When the pet slips outside, you have no idea where the pet has been—or what it might bring inside. Several cases of rabies have been reported in humans. Do not let yourself be one of the statistics of death by rabies.

Top Human Medications Poisonous to Pets

If you know which human drugs are harmful to pets, you can take steps to prevent these compounds from being placed where pets can reach them. According to the Pet Poison Helpline, the following are the top causes of toxicity in pets due to human medications:

- *Non-Steroid Anti-Inflammatory Drugs (Advil, Aleve, Motrin)*: These are harmful to your pet if even one or two tablets are consumed. The compounds cause serious stomach and intestinal ulcers and kidney failure.
- *Acetaminophen (Tylenol):* In cats, acetaminophen causes damage to red blood cells, which limits the ability to carry oxygen to tissues, creating asphyxiation. In dogs, acetaminophen results in liver failure and, in large doses, red blood cell damage.
- *Antidepressants (Effexor, Cymbalta, Prozac, Lexapro):* Although some of these are used in pets under a doctor's order, overdoses by pet owners lead to serious neurological problems, sedation, loss of coordination, tremors, and seizures. Some antidepressants cause

elevated heart rates, increased blood pressure, and elevated body temperatures.

- *Attention-Deficit Disorder and Attention-Deficit Hyperactivity Disorder Medications:* Small amounts cause life-threatening tremors, seizures, elevated body temperatures, and heat problems. Make sure these drugs are not out so that your pet accidently gets to them. Be safety conscious.

- *Benzodiazepines and Sleep Aids (Xanax, Klonopin, Ambien, Lunesta):* Unfortunately, these compounds create hyperactivity, hyper-excitement, and agitation in pets. They also cause severe lethargy, loss of coordination, and slow respiration. In cats, benzodiazepines can cause liver failure.

- *Birth Control Medications (Estrogen, Estradiol, Progesterone):* Small amount in pets are not normally a problem. Unless the package was almost empty, the pet can overdose. Large overdoses cause bone marrow suppression. All the blood cells are made in the bone marrow. If the bone marrow is severely depressed, the pet can die from lack of blood or anemia. The bone marrow can also become severely damaged.

- *Angiotensin-Converting Enzyme or ACE Inhibitors (Zestril, Altace):* These compounds are used to treat high blood pressure and are sometimes are prescribed by veterinarians for pet use. Pets that happen to get into human prescription medications tend to eat way too much of the drug, causing an overdosing that lowers blood pressure and causes dizziness and weakness. If small amounts of these compounds are ingested, home monitoring can be accomplished—unless the pet has kidney failure or heart disease. As with any human medicine, it is important to prevent your pet from getting to these compounds unintentionally. A little caution can prevent a lot of heartburn and sadness.

- *Beta-Blockers (Tenormin, Toprol, Coreg):* Small amounts can cause life-threatening blood pressure drops and slowed heart rates. These compounds need to be kept securely away from pets. Many times, owners are away when pets ingest human compounds, giving lots of time for the drugs to have an effect. An owner can find a dead pet or a pet very near death. Keep human drugs away from pets.
- *Thyroid Hormones (Armour, Synthroid):* Dogs with an underactive thyroid need larger doses than people do. If a dog happens to get into thyroid medications, it is usually not an issue. However, large overdoses of thyroid medications cause muscle tremors, nervousness, panting, rapid heart rates, and aggression in dogs and cats.
- *Cholesterol-Lowering Agents or Statins (Lipitor, Zocor, Crestor):* Fortunately, these compounds normally only cause mild vomiting or diarrhea. Serious problems only occur from long-term use.

The following are safety tips to help prevent pets from becoming poisoned by human drugs:

Never leave loose pills in a plastic Ziploc bag. It is too easy for a pet to destroy the bag and get to the medicines.

If you use a weekly medicine container, keep it where a pet cannot get to it. Pets are a very capable of opening them.

Do not store human medicines with pet medicines because you might mix them up. In case you were wondering, it is not a good idea for you to take pet medications.

Children's medicines are not necessarily safe for pets. Keep them separated.

There are many poison centers. Here are some telephone numbers for quick reference in case of an emergency:

Pet Poison Helpline 1-800-213-6680 (consultation fee is $35). The ASPCA poison number is 1-800-426-4435 (consultation fee is $65). Your state may have a poison center. Some veterinary colleges have a toxicology department that you may contact with your pet's toxicities. Also, your pet's doctor is a great resource during emergencies.

Sore Mouth Due to Loose Teeth

Many conditions cause pets to have a sore mouth. These include bacterial infections, chicken bones caught between the teeth and buried deep in the tissues in the roof of the mouth, sore teeth, and many others. These common conditions can cause oral drooling and weight loss.

Sometimes a mouth can appear normal when the owner looks inside. However, the pet stops eating almost as soon as the food goes in the mouth. It is obvious that the pet wants to eat, but there are obvious signs of pain.

The cause of this is often a sore loose tooth that is causing pain. The most common teeth involved are the anterior incisor teeth. Carefully attempt to move each tooth back and forth with slight pressure. When the painful tooth is discovered, the dog will react—and you will know which tooth is causing the problem. Since there is always a chance that more than one tooth is involved, attempt to move other teeth. Once the problem tooth is identified, it can easily be treated.

Treatment:

Simply remove the tooth. Even though you may have been able to move it back and forth, a solid pull might be required to remove the tooth. Do not break the tooth. Pull the entire tooth up or down with one quick jerk. Be aware that tooth removal is painful. We have special tools for this procedure. I have not used household pliers, but they should work if you are able to get a good grip on the tooth. Another option is to let a doctor pull the tooth.

Prevention:

Allowing the dog to chew on hard objects is the most common cause of this syndrome. Chewing on hard items helps eliminate tartar on the teeth, but they can cause trauma in the mouth.

Dandruff or Scaling or Crusting

Dandruff is a sign of a health condition, but it is not a disease or a condition that stands alone. What is the cause of dandruff in your pet? There are numerous causes—from simple to very complex. You can do some simple things to help with dandruff, scaling, or crusting.

Dandruff is present on the skin as large flakes. Crusts may be composed of thick scales, pus, blood, serum, or other pus-producing organisms. These conditions are usually secondary.

There is definitely a difference in cats and dog. Cats are normally not affected, but dogs may have a skin infection. Age and the type of skin parasite—some can infect people—play a role. Conditions or parasites that make the pet scratch or pruritus can cause dandruff in dogs or cats.

The following are some of the causes of dandruff: bacterial skin infections, fungal infections, parasitic infections, allergies, viral skin infections, endocrine problems, Cushing's disease, and congenital, hereditary, environmental, and nutritional issues. Dandruff can have a very serious cause.

The most common causes of dandruff are bacterial infections of the skin and fleas. If you see scales with hair holes in them, it is a sign of a skin bacterial infection common in cats. Some cats have scaling when the humidity is low in winter due to heating the home. Scabies can cause excessive and severe dandruff. Cats that cannot groom show more dandruff than those that can groom. In dogs, fleas and demodex are common.

As a general rule, cats and dogs that go outside get skin parasites. Older dogs and cats get skin cancers or immune-mediated diseases. These conditions are more frequent in certain breeds. The three most common causes of dandruff are fleas, skin fungal infections, and yeast infections, which can be quite extensive in dogs. Bacterial skin infections are most common in cats.

Treatment:

In some cases, low humidity of a heated home can be the cause of dandruff. Take this into consideration—and do not treat things that are not present in or on the pet. I recommend Advantage II for cats and small dogs and Advantix II for dogs. Both are very effective and kill fleas, flea larvae, and flea eggs. Demodex can be treated with Ivermectin. (See below to determine the dosage of Ivermectin for treating demodex mange mite). Flea medications are applied on the back of the neck every month. Ivermectin for demodex is given orally. Demodex treatment can require up to six months, but the disease usually clears within one or two months. Flea medications can be purchased at military instillations at either the BX or PX, Petco, PetSmart, and feed stores. It can also be found in some Wal-Mart stores.

How to Calculate Ivermectin Dosage for Demodex Mange:

Warning: do not use these calculations unless your pet weighs twenty-five pounds. This example shows how to calculate the proper dose for your pet based on its weight. Please double-check your math before administering the drug. Let's use a twenty-five-pound dog in this example:

- For Day 1, divide the weight of the dog in pounds by 100. 25 pounds/100 =.25 cc. On Day 1, the dose is .25 cc (only 1/4 of a cc or ml).
- On Day 2, double the Day 1 dosage. The Day 2 dosage would be .50 cc (1/2 cc or ml only).
- On Days 3–14, double the Day 2 dose so that the dose (1 cc) is given daily for the next twelve days.

Prevention:

The underlying causes of dandruff are complex. Not all causes can be treated with over-the-counter drugs. Monthly treatment for fleas goes a long way in preventing a major source of dandruff. Constantly be aware of your pet's health. It helps to start a wellness program with your pet's doctor and have exams every six months or once a year at a minimum.

Cat Ear Infestation and Infection Due to Demodex

Demodex is not common in the ears I have treated. However, if you treat what is believed to be a usual ear mite infestation with the typical ear mite (*Otodectes cynotis*) and it does not resolve or get well, the cat may have an infection caused by demodex mites. There is no difference in appearance of the ear with demodex compared with the traditional ear mite infestation.

After a swab is inserted into the ear to obtain some of the ear materials, the material is placed under a microscope to identify the parasite. If you do not have a microscope, you can follow the treatment below. If it is a persistent demodex ear infestation, you will clear the demodex infestation.

Treatment:

If you have tried to treat what you believe to be a normal ear parasite infestation and it does not resolve, you can try this treatment. You will need Ivermectin—just as with the normal ear mite infestation. You can purchase Ivermectin at any feed or tractor store. Simply clean the ears, apply one half milliliter (cc) of Ivermectin every day into the ear, and massage the ears well. Continue this treatment until you do not see any more materials in the ear.

Continue with one half milliliter (cc) of Ivermectin in the ears every day for two weeks. If you stop too soon, you will not kill the demodex mites. Be sure to finish the job. An ear infestation of yeast can appear just like a mite infestation; be aware if a microscope diagnosis is not made.

Prevention:

Check your cat's ears frequently by looking into them. Since the ear canal bends, it is not possible to see beyond the bend without an ear scope (otoscope). If you see an accumulation of materials (sometimes black and brown), suspect the start of an ear infection or an infestation of ear mites.

Chapter 6:
Other Issues of Importance
for Dogs and Cats

*Moral courage is the most valuable and usually
the most absent characteristic in man.*
—*George S. Patton*

This chapter has some interesting things that affect pets. Not all are medical, but they are important for providing health care to your pets. You will understand what information is obtained when a CBC and blood chemistry is completed. An awareness is essential to know the effects of stress some pets can experience when confronted with a new or different environment. This author knows of pets that have been euthanized just because the owner did not understand simple pet stress of a new environment. You are always confronted with administrative issues that go along with ownership and responsibility of our little dog and cat buddies.

Identifying Pain in Pets

Pain occurs in all animals. It is an unpleasant feeling or emotional experience that may be associated with tissue damage, such as kidney disease, liver damage, broken bones, or muscle trauma. Differences in age, sex, breeding lines, and species can alter responses to different types of pain. The responses to pain vary greatly; there is no set list of signs that are always present.

The most common or recognizable signs of pain in dogs and cats include vocalization, agitation, abnormal posture or gait, thrashing, sensitivity to touch, being supersensitive to painful stimulation, or responding to normally nonpainful stimulation. Chronic pain from kidney pain, tumors, pancreatitis, hip dysplasia, arthritis, or other systemic diseases can result in not eating, reduced activity, lameness, or depression.

Treatment:

Treatment depends on the source and type of pain. Pain is a condition that should be assessed by your pet's doctor. Identifying and treating the cause of the pain is the only way to eliminate the pain. Nonsteroid pain relievers aid—but do not treat—the cause of pain. Aspirin can kill cats because cats cannot metabolize aspirin. Aspirin is not going to help kidney damage or pancreatic disease, but it may benefit acute pains, such as being hit by a car, broken bones, or dog bites.

As with any disease process, the cause of the condition must be treated to eliminate the signs and stop the pain. One cannot treat the signs and expect resolution of the pain associated with any disease process because the disease or condition must be treated. Dogs can be treated with aspirin with a dose of 4 mg to 10 mg per pound of body weight given every twelve hours. Aspirin comes in 81 mg and 325 mg tablets.

The goal with pain treatment is to use the lowest possible dose that will provide the best pain relief. As a general rule, one-fourth of a 325 mg aspirin per ten pounds can be given as a pain dose. The charts below will provide you with a dose by weight to use for treating your dog. Remember that cats should not receive aspirin.

Since aspirin comes in tablet form as either 81 mg or 325 mg, it has to be cut into quarters. You may have to give only a quarter of a tablet or perhaps a tablet or two and a quarter or a half to get close to the necessary dosage. It is impossible with the tablets available to get accurate doses of aspirin. However, we can get close. In some cases, the chart shows a little less than the actual calculated dose (and some a little more) due to the size of the tablets available.

Dog Aspirin Dose Chart
Aspirin Is Not Recommend for Cats
Use Enteric-Coated Aspirin

Caution Special Notice: Anything Under Five Pounds Should Have a Prescription from the Pet's Doctor

(Give Every Twelve Hours)

Weight Pounds	Low Dose 4.5 Mg /Pd 81 Mg Tablet	High Dose 11 Mg Tablet 325 Mg Tablet	Weight Pounds	Low Dose 4.5 Mg /Pd 325 Mg Tablet	High Dose 11 Mg Tablet 325 Mg Tablet	Weight Pounds	Low Dose 81 Mg Tablet 4.5 Mg /Pd	High Dose 11 Mg Tablet 325 Mg Tablet
5	.25	.25	26	.25	1	46	.75	1+.5
6	.25	.25	27	.25	1	47	.75	1+.5
7	.25	.25	28	.25	1	48	.75	1+.5
8	.5	.25	29	.25	1	49	.75	1+.5
9	.5	.25	30	.5	1	50	.75	1+.75
10	.5	.25	31	.5	1	51	.75	1+.75
11	.5	.5	32	.5	1+.25	52	.75	1+.75
12	.5	.5	33	.5	1+.25	53	.75	1+.75
13	.75	.5	34	.5	1+.25	54	.75	2
14	.75	.5	35	.5	1+.25	55	.75	2
15	.75	.5	36	.5	1+.25	56	.75	2
16	.75	.5	37	.5	1+.25	57	.75	2
17	1	.5	38	.5	1+.25	58	.75	2
18	1	.5	39	.5	1+.25	59	.75	2
19	1	.75	40	.5	1+.5	60	.75	2
20	1	.75	41	.5	1+.5	61	.75	2

Weight Pounds	Low Dose 4.5 Mg /Pd 325 Mg Tablet	High Dose 11 Mg Tablet 325 Mg Tablet
21	25	75
22	25	75
23	25	75
24	25	75
42	5	1+5
43	5	1+5
44	5	1+5
45	5	1+5
62	.75	2
63	1	2
64	1	2
65	1	2
66	1	2+.25
67	1	2+.25
68	1	2+.25
69	1	2+.25
70	1	2+.5
71	1	2+.5
72	1	2+.5
73	1	2+.5
74	1	2+.5
75	1	2+.5
76	1	2+.5
77	1	2+.5
78	1	2+.75
79	1	2+.75
80	1+.25	2+.75
81	1+.25	2+.75
82	1+.25	2+.75
83	1+.25	3
84	1+.25	3
85	1+.25	3
86	1+.25	3
87	1+.25	3
88	1+.25	3
89	1+.25	3
90	1+.25	3
91	1+.25	3+.25
92	1+.25	3+.25
93	1+.25	3+.25
94	1+.25	3+.25
95	1+.25	3+.25
96	1+.25	3+.25
97	1+.25	3+.25
98	1+.5	3+.25
99	1+.5	3+.25
100	1+.5	3+.5

Prevention:

No one can predict the future, but one can aid a pet's health with having routine health checks. Wellness programs for people and pets have proven their worth in financial savings and in preventing health conditions due to early diagnosis. Healthy pets do not have pain. One of the major pain producers is letting pets get hit by cars; this can be avoided by keeping pets on a leash and being with the pet during outings.

Hairy Pets and Hot Summers

If you live in a warm climate and you have a pet with lots of hair, the heat may be more than a hairy dog can handle comfortably. Is it appropriate to clip the hair in the summer to aid the pet with the heat?

Treatment:

This is a personal decision, but it seems logical that if one tries to comfort the pet in very hot weather, it would seem prudent to clip the hair of the pet. The bottom line in this phenomenon is that hair grows back. The only reason one would not clip the hair in very hot environments is if they believe that the look of the clipped pet is too goofy.

I have noted that when the pet is first clipped, the pet tends to look a little goofy or strange. In time, the short hair is not even noticeable—and it certainly helps the pet handle hot weather. The Furminator removes dead hairs very effectively. It is a bit expensive, but its effectiveness overcomes the cost. If you obtain a Furminator, you will be pleased with its operation. Furminators are available at pet stores.

Prevention:

Unfortunately, many pets with longer hair have many matted hair masses that are unsightly and allow dirt, grime, and skin infections to accumulate. Matted hair can easily be prevented by using a Furminator frequently, clipping the hair, and keeping the pet properly groomed. Keep the coat clean and properly groomed.

Identification Method for Your Pet

People tell me all the time that a pet is a very important part of the family. When a pet gets lost, the owner has to find it. Our facility has hundreds of cats and dogs that not a soul has attempted to locate. However, when the animal has appropriate identification, we have been able to return the pet to the rightful owner.

What is the best identification available? What can other identification methods do? First and foremost, of course no identification is the worst. It shows a lack of forethought. Many pets that never go outside have no identification. However, many of these get out—and get lost because they have no sense of direction. In the treatment section, I will rank many ID methods. Be aware that any ID is far better than no ID at all.

Treatment:

Identification chips have become quite popular. They seem to be the best method for finding the owner. If the owner does not register the chip, it is useless. Chips do not fall off the pet because they are implanted under the skin.

Identification tags have the name, address, and telephone number of the owner. Unfortunately, tags of any sort can become separated from the pet or its collar.

After an identification tag, a rabies tag can be useful in tracking down an owner. The bottom of the list is no identification of any form. Be a friend of your pet and get a chip or an identification tag of some sort. The pet that is returned may be your own.

Prevention:

We see so many pets that could be returned to their owners if they only had some sort of identification on them. Lack of identification can be the cause of euthanasia. Identification can be the difference between the return of your pet and never seeing the pet again.

Signs and pictures on bulletin boards do not get pets home; it takes identification on the pet. Do not put it off—do it now.

Pet Insurance

Pet insurance is much more prevalent and available in this age of veterinary medicine than ever before. To insure a pet is a personal decision—just like any other type of insurance. Many folks with insurance have been pleased with the product—especially when their pets have had health issues.

There are all kinds of opportunities for issues just as with any type of insurance. I have no bias toward any company. Each insurance carrier has multiple insurance plans to choose from. If it were not for the insurance coverage, some pets would have had to be euthanized due to projected costs. In those instances, insurance has saved the lives of pets.

Treatment:

Pet insurance covers several types of injuries: poisoning, trauma, immunization reactions, hypothyroid issues, and many other issues. Pet insurance companies can be found online; on their websites, you can learn about the products they provide. Having pet insurance is a personal decision for the pet owner. It is easy to find insurance carriers online by searching for pet insurance.

Transient Stress Syndrome or Von Gierke-Like Syndrome

This syndrome is most often brought on by a trip to the veterinary hospital for immunizations. When the pet arrives home, the pet seems lethargic, reluctant to move, and not playful. Many folks ask what they can do when they observe this syndrome. This is normally due to a Von Gierke-like syndrome or transient stress. The stress of the trip to the veterinary hospital—and the vaccines—causes the dog to burn excess sugars, resulting in the Von Gierke-like syndrome.

Treatment:

Giving the pet a tablespoon or two of Karo syrup will often bring the pet out of the stupor rather quickly. I have had folks tell me how this treatment worked; many are astounded that the dog came around so fast. Others reported that it had no effect at all. If it works for your pet—great. If not, it is a matter of waiting it out. It is not a major concern if it does not work.

Prevention:

The simple treatment of transient stress or Von Gierke-like syndrome is Karo syrup. If your pet has this issue, try giving the syrup twenty or thirty minutes before departing. It does not hurt to give more syrup when you return home. See how it goes because the treatment works in some and not in others.

The Story of Blood Tests

The most common blood tests that doctors order involve two major parameters that tend to reveal the health of your pet. These tests cannot be foretold by looking at—or feeling—the pet. These tests allow modern medicine to be accomplished. The two major tests are the complete blood count and the blood chemistry. These two tests evaluate your pet's health and give a background on the interpretation of organ systems that are in trouble. It is not hieroglyphics, and you can understand them. Other special tests that will not be covered include thyroid function tests, biopsies, and Cushing's testing.

Complete Blood Count

- *A complete blood count* usually includes a red cell count, a white cell count, hematocrit, hemoglobin, platelet count, and some red blood cell indices.

- *Red blood cells:* Red blood cells carry oxygen to other parts of the body. They also carry carbon dioxide back to the lungs so it can be exhaled while breathing. A shortage of red cells indicates anemia, and too many red cells might indicate a blood cancer.

- *Hematocrit (packed cell volume)* is a measure of the space or volume that the red cells take up in the blood. The value is given as a percentage; the average is about 45 percent. A low percentage is a sign of anemia; one that is too high indicates dehydration or a blood cancer.

- *Hemoglobin* is in the red cells. This compound carries oxygen and carbon dioxide. A normal hemoglobin level is about 15 percent. It measures oxygenation of body tissues.

- *Red blood cell indices* measure the size of the red cells and the amount of hemoglobin in each cell.

- *White blood cells*: Sometimes the white cell count is referred to as a leukocyte count. These cells are the protectors against infections. These cells attack and kill bacteria, viruses, and other organisms that cause infections. If the white cells are unable to kill, the infections will persist. Your pet may need antibiotics to help the cells destroy the invading organisms.

- White blood cells come in a variety of cells that have similar functions. They attack invading organisms and different types of invaders. Just as an army of soldiers has different functions, white cells have different functions. They still attack and destroy infectious organisms. The major players are neutrophils (attackers of bacteria) and lymphocytes (attackers of viruses). *Eosinophils* and *basophils* are interested in parasites and muscle infections (eosinophilic myositis). Each type of cell will normally increase with different types of infections, depending on the specific need for cells to attack different infectious agents. Too many immature cells may indicate leukemia.

- *Platelets* are the smallest type of blood cell. They are important for blood clotting. When bleeding occurs, the platelets clump together to form a sticky plug that helps to stop bleeding.

Blood Chemistry

There are different varieties of blood chemistry tests, and not every machine will complete the same tests. Different labs have slightly different values for normal, and some blood chemistries have more or less items. A typical blood chemistry panel will include:

1. General Metabolism
   Glucose (GLU)
   Lactate Dehydrogenase (LDH)
   Creatine Phosphokinase (CPK)

2. Kidney Function
   Blood Urea Nitrogen (BUN)
   Creatinine (CREAT)

3. Liver Function
   Alkaline Phosphatase (ALP)
   Albumin (ALB)
   Gamma-Glutamyl Transpeptidase (GGT)
   Alanine Aminotransferase (ALT)
   Total Protein (TP)
   Cholesterol (CHOL)
   Globulin (GLOB)
   Total Bilirubin (TBILI)

4. Thyroid
>   Triiodothyronine (T3)
>   Thyroxine (T4)

5. Pancreas
>   Amylase (AMY)
>   Lipase (LIP)

Treatment:

The test results allow your pet's doctor to decide what needs to be done to help cure the pet. Without these tests, there is no way to know what is wrong—or which organ system is the cause of the health condition being presented for treatment.

Prevention:

Be sure to have a biannual checkup or start a wellness plan for your pet. A wellness plan allows for early diagnosis and treatment that may not be treatable if left until a condition is advanced. In veterinary medicine, prevention means a healthy pet. It is much cheaper to prevent disease than to treat it.

American Veterinary Medical Association

The American Veterinary Medical Association (AVMA) has a website that provides information about preventive health care, food safety and recalls, first-aid tips, post-vaccination expectations, safe use of flea and tick products, emergency and disaster preparedness information, how to select a veterinarian, and a lot more. To get to the website, enter AVMA on the search line and American Veterinary Medical Association pops up. Select this entry or enter www.avma.org and the AVMA website will open. At the top of the page, click on "Animal Health." Scroll down the page to the topic you would like to learn about. In no event shall the American Veterinary Medical Association be liable for any special, incidental, indirect, or consequential damages of any kind arising out of or in connection with the use of the publications or other material posted on its website, whether or not advised of the possibility of such damages, and on any theory of liability.

A New Home for Your Cat

It is not uncommon for families to get a new cat when they get a new home. This often causes the cat to become reclusive. It may hide somewhere in the house and not come out to explore its new environment. This is not a disease—it is a normal fear in the cat. It takes time for a cat to adjust to a new environment. Be patient with the cat. Cats that hide when company or strangers visit are most prone to having a difficult time adjusting to a new environment.

Treatment:

Be patient. Let the cat adjust to the new home or environment. Put the cat into one room with the litter, food, and water. Normally, in due time, the cat will start to explore the remainder of the house. Soon it will become a normal member of the family. The process of adjusting to the new home or environment may take a month or more.

Prevention:

Patience is the name of the game with the change to a new home or getting a new cat into a new environment. The onus of prevention is on the owner. He or she may start to think that the cat has a health problem, but it is usually fear. In time, the cat will be fine.

About the Author

Dr. Robert Ridgway graduated from Kansas State University College of Veterinary Medicine and completed a residency in Internal Medicine at the University of California, Davis. After graduating from veterinary college, he worked for a short period of time at a veterinary hospital in Topeka, Kansas. He entered the US Army Veterinary Corps, where he became director of the Animal Medicine Division on Okinawa. He later completed a residency of comparative medicine at the Madigan Army Medical Center. He is a graduate of Officer Candidate School at Fort Sill, Oklahoma, and a graduate of the US Army Command and General Staff College. He was the treasurer of the District of Columbia Academy of Veterinary Medicine for fourteen years. He served as secretary-treasurer and president of the District of Columbia Veterinary Medical Association. He was the first US Army officer to be in charge of the Department of Defense Military Dog Veterinary Service at Lackland Air Force Base in San Antonio, Texas. He completed a master's of international management at the University of Maryland, University College. After retiring from the army, he worked at Covance Laboratories and Banfield Pet Hospital. He is currently employed at Orange County Animal Services in Orlando, Florida. Dr. Ridgway is a diplomate in the American College of Preventive Medicine and a diplomate in the College of Laboratory Animal Medicine. Dr. Ridgway is married and has one daughter and one male cat.

Index

The following blank pages are for recording the following:

Dates of visits to the veterinary clinic (immunizations, titer checks, treatments, surgery, etc.)

Health checks at home (heart rate, temperature, respiration, heart sounds, etc.)

Your treatment of your pet, date of treatment, what you treated with, dosage, and number of days you gave the treatment

Number of puppies or kittens born, date, and any issues with birth

Exams of puppies or kittens

Health and treatment of puppies or kittens, sick young, etc., including drugs used

Number of the litter that died

Any other events you want to record

CPSIA information can be obtained at www.ICGtesting.com
Printed in the USA
LVOW05s1623020114

367797LV00020B/966/P

9 781469 775258